Saving Face

The Scents-Able Way
to Wrinkle-Free Skin

Natural, Green Beauty Secrets

Using Essential Oils—No Toxic Chemicals

*Christine Arceneaux
'2017
Young Living
Beauty School, Canada*

Sabina M. DeVita, Ed.D., N.N.C.P.

A PUBLICATION OF

The Wellness Institute of Living and Learning

NEW REVISED 3rd EDITION

JULY 2016 A.D.

2nd edition JULY 2003 A.D

NEW REVISED 3rd EDITION

JULY 2016

Wellness Institute of Living and Learning
7700 Hurontario St., Suite 408
Brampton, ON L6Y 4M3
Canada · 905-451-4475
www.savingfacescentsably.com

Original Cover Design by Stewart Publishing Company

New Cover design by VirtualGraphicArtsDepartment.com

Formatting by DocUmeant Designs

Cover Caption: One of the most famous faces in the world is that of the graceful and exquisite Queen Nefertiti as seen in this 3350-year-old sculpture sculpture on page xvii. She was the wife of Akhenaton, who ruled Egypt 1375–1358 B.C. Appropriately; her name means: "The beautiful woman has come". Egyptian Queens such as Nefertiti, Hatshepsut (1502–1482 B.C.) and Cleopatra (69–30 B.C.) all maintained their beauty and youthful appearances by applying and bathing in essential oils and using other natural products.

DEDICATION

This book is dedicated to the empowering of the female spirit—free of suffering, pain, victim-hood and avoid-able cancer and other diseases.

May all of you who search for Beauty and Longevity be filled with truth, love, enlightenment, freedom to be and inner knowing of who you truly are.

CONTENTS

FOREWORD

BY MARY YOUNG
Executive Vice President of Young Living Company

It has been a long time since I have read such a comprehensive book about skin care that is concise, easy to understand with a simple, practical application. Almost everyone is concerned about feeling and looking better. Practically every magazine and newspaper is filled with "fantastic" remedies, "secret" potions and lotions with "amazing" cures and "wonder" results. Television commercials are an irritation as they interrupt programs to promote more "cures" or "potions"; billboards stare us in the face as we drive down the road advertising more toxic products.

We rarely read the label because we can't pronounce the words or our eyes skip to just the "active" ingredients touted on the label. With the vast amount of toxic poisonous substances listed as natural ingredients, the unaware public will continue to wonder why they are tired, lethargic, confused, unhealthy and aging.

In my personal relationship with Dr. Sabina DeVita, I have found an individual who is extremely well educated, who is constantly studying and doing research, who is driven to find out the "why" and know the truth or that which she pursues.

> With the vast amount of toxic poisonous substances listed as natural ingredients, the unaware public will continue to wonder why they are tired, lethargic, confused, unhealthy and aging.

I have been interested in health and longevity my entire life. My husband, Gary, has devoted his life to holistic healing and lives and walks today because of his intense desire to find the natural substances our creator has given us to achieve vibrant health. We are passionate about our quest to understand God's laws and his direction for our spiritual and physical well-being. I find that Sabina has embraced the same philosophy for truth and health with similar tenacity as Gary and myself. Essential oils are a great blessing to us and for those who choose to embrace this knowledge.

Sabina has brought the complexity of such vast information into a very succinct and simple language, and brings tremendous knowledge and insight to her writing from which we all may benefit. Her remedies and formulas are interesting and creative, and anyone can have fun experimenting. In the world of "natural," only your body knows and you have to let your body find out what it likes and wants.

I express my respect and love for the immense time and dedication that Sabina has given to write this book for those seeking truth and enlightenment. May we all work together sharing knowledge, uplifting one another, and living life with joy and fulfillment.

PREFACE

More than ever before in our history, we are living in a most 'toxic' chemical world with monumental demands in our daily lives. The heightened desire for youth, long healthy lives, beauty, agility and vibrancy has been fed and manipulated for years by media hype, fake promises, trickery, poisonous consumables and glamorous ads.

Unfortunately, there are too many who are not aware that the unregulated cosmetic and personal care industry has left us with a complex chemical soup that is devastating to our lives and our planet, all too often in the name of beauty. I discovered through my own suffering from environmental allergies and chemical sensitivities how toxic these personal care products were. It became important for me to use (and first find) organic, clean, pure personal care products, cosmetics, household cleaners, food and water. I was forced to change my total lifestyle as I was experiencing a number of severe reactions such as: brain fog, fatigue, depression, headaches, red burning eyes, inability to concentrate, sleepiness, red itchy skin and nervousness.

My reactions to all household and personal skin care products and other indoor environmental pollutants became a relentless issue for me, hampering my way of life completely. Car fumes caused severe drowsiness to the point that I couldn't drive as I fought to stay awake while driving. Many times I would stop on the side of the road to sleep. I stopped purchasing personal care chemical products, be it soap, shampoo, lipstick, detergents etc. as I reacted to them in so many ways (as listed above) including their negative impact on my emotions and moods. I became quite sensitive to items in my home as well, such as, the natural gas heating system (most severe), wall to wall carpets, particle board cupboards and so on.

Since conventional medicine could only offer me their anti-histamine toxic drugs and allergy injections, which were making me worse, I turned my attention to natural health methods for my own healing. This led me to researching what was then a new

ment will inspire you to do more in the world, not only in personal care and beauty but in other areas in your lives and businesses as well. You too can become someone that can

phenomenon: called environmental illness, or 20th century disease. I discovered how toxic our world had become with ecological toxins, chemical inhalants, pollutants, smog, electromagnetic pollution and chemical poisons in our foods, products, water and air.

I left my position as a guidance counselor and teacher at the time, to pursue a doctoral degree in psychology specializing in brain allergies (a term I learned from psychiatrist Dr. Philpott), a rare combination scarcely known or considered for mental health issues—even to this day. "Brain Allergies" are rarely regarded as a major factor in our mental and emotional well-being. Since I was experiencing this debilitating 'phenomenon' myself, I knew it was important to research and understand it further. How many people were and are also 'ill' especially from their environmental toxic overload only to be mis-diagnosed for mental illness and prescribed something more toxic that never addresses the real underlying issues?

My university doctorate became the first work of its kind in the field of psychology at the University of Toronto—in fact, it was the first of its kind on 'brain allergies' and in environmental or ecological sciences in psychology. In the years that followed, I became involved with a number of environmental groups: supporting them in their pursuit for cleaner and safer environments, personal care and household products, to protect endangered species, conserve wild plant life and literally protect and preserve ourselves.

Due to my holistic energy—medicine studies, research and personal experiences in my own healing, I felt it was important to open a private practice to help others in the understanding of the BRAIN—Body, Mind and Spirit inter-relatedness. I have been offering my services for the past 28 years, utilizing cutting-edge energy healing practices and energy technologies. I sourced the finest organic, safe, whole-natured botanicals, herbs and healing products. In the late 1990s, I discovered the power of organic, genuine, 'therapeutic' quality Grade-A essential oils and the art and science of French medicinal aromatherapy. These precious and live, super-food essential oils were very different. I then introduced them into my practice and into all of my natural healing classes. As I continued to add to my holistic healing modalities, I became involved in skin care utilizing a micro-circulation/color/gemstone technology along with the essential oils. I learned that the acupressure face points were a doorway to the rest of the body's organs.

I realized how crucial it was then and still is today that you know how the chemicals in our everyday lives and in our personal care products influence our well-being on all levels as well as how toxic they are to our environment and our skin. Beauty, health and longevity are interconnected. This book will guide you to learn to become beautiful, vibrant, healthy and young in a safe, whole and ecological way on your own. Hopefully, this self-empowerment will inspire you to do more in the world, not only in personal care and beauty but in other areas in your lives and businesses as well. You too can become someone that can help create a better peaceful world. We know that happy, well, vibrant people are more able to help make the world a better and peaceful place. Let's Face it, isn't that what we all desire on our planet? Now you have an added advantage, that is, you can feel and look healthier and younger too!

I believe that knowledge is the key to freedom and most importantly, knowledge that is acted upon brings about power, healing and transformations.

Over the years, in my holistic private practice, I listened to many women complain of various ailments, emotional stresses, their traumas, their toxic emotions and skin related problems. Too many of my clients were not aware of what these toxic, harmful chemicals, used topically and in their housecleaning products, were doing to their health on a daily basis; nor was I until I became ill.

> . . . knowledge that is acted upon brings about power, healing and transformations.

This book is also meant to be a hands-on, simple, natural guide to skin care using **real-green aromatic essential oils**. Being healthy and beautiful is not only learning to avoid the toxins but also learning how to feed and nurture your largest vital organ, your skin: plus learning to nurture all your body organs and your mind with Live Super foods.

It is not a surprise that natural skin care is more than skin deep—it starts with good health on the inside, which this guidebook addresses as well. Currently, the advances in the anti-aging movement are bringing about a tremendous awareness in utilizing a more natural approach to preventing the signs of aging. We have, more than ever before, the means to maintain optimum health and beautiful, youthful skin. But the challenge is to know what is healthy and available or become enamored and confused with the imposters.

Please congratulate yourself for purchasing **Saving Face** and your willingness to learn to use Mother Nature's most powerful, natural, wholesome nutrients and precious gifts on your skin. You have the answers in your hands and the means to slow down the biological clock. It's totally up to you—You make the choices in what you use, eat, drink and slather on your face.

Over the years in observing the results from conducting several Aroma Facial-at-home-Spa workshops, it became quite clear to me how powerful these essential oils are on so many levels of health and skin care for both women and men.

While essential oils can be used in a variety of ways, even for electromagnetic smog (see my book on **Electromagnetic Pollution** (www.electromagneticpollution.net) and household 'Green' cleaning and brain, pineal health (www.vibrationalcleaning.com) this book is focused primarily on skin and The FACE! *Saving Face* also presents many breakthroughs of several 'anti-aging' discoveries along with essential oils usage and health benefits.

My personal study of aromatics for mental-emotional health care has awakened a deeper reverence for me for Mother Nature's inherent wisdom and versatility. Today, these essential oils play a vital part in my life. Every day, in some way, I use these precious essential oils (see my preference below from the Young Living Company for their wild-crafted or organic—chemical free oils—also read more in chapter 6). I use them:

- in my shower for my hair and skin;
- on my face to keep it moisturized, nourished and youthful;
- as my underarm deodorant;
- to keep me focused;
- to remain calm during times of stress;
- to support my immune system;
- to balance my hormones;
- to purify my indoor air
- in all of my household cleaning.
- in my food preparations and
- to create insect deterrent sprays and to soothe my skin

MY CHOICE IN COMPANIES

Just a brief word as to why I chose the Young Living essential oils Company as my primary and only choice in using or recommending essential oils. I know that there are very few small and private companies that produce high quality essential oils in the world and it is a matter of sourcing them. Young Living's essential oils fit perfectly for what I wanted in a product due to their authenticity and guarantee that they are pure, 100% chemical free (no solvents in distillation either), wild-crafted or organically grown by sustainable and ecological farming practices: that is, they use absolutely no pesticides, herbicides, fungicides or agricultural chemicals of any kind in cultivating and in distilling their crops. What a treasure it was for me to find Young Living, a solid 20 year old company today who has built a pres-tigious reputation as well as building many of their own global farms. Some companies have now even mimicked Young Living—using similar messages and formulations—so consum-ers beware. I finally found essential oils that I did not react to; could trust, apply on my skin, breathe and even ingest them. These essential oils are being used for healing purposes, even in hospitals today, thus their original descriptive word "therapeutic".

D. Gary Young founder of Young Living Company plus grower, harvester and distiller of the Young Living crops, starts with nurturing the soil before planting by using a combination of minerals, organic mulch, manure and enzymes. Today, Young Living owns and operates the largest privately owned organic herb farms in the world now in 9 countries, 12 farms and upholds the prominent seal of "Seed to Seal" distinction in the aromatherapy, essential oil industry. They have shown to have one of the highest standards in the world. All their oil samples are sent to two or up to five independent laboratories for testing, to be sure that they conform to the International (ISO) and (AFNOR) standards for therapeutic-grade essential oils.

the essential oil quality as nature provided is everything in achieving the desired results of health and glowing, radiant skin.

But even more powerfully, Young Living has set their own high standards of excellence and purity giving a new meaning to genuine, therapeutic grade essential oils—matter of fact, D. Gary Young coined the term 'therapeutic' grade essential oils' back in early 2004. This term was never used beforehand until the founder's unrivaled expertise on the therapeutic power of plants as well as his impeccable standards for high quality led to the creation of the world's largest line of genuine, therapeutic essential oils and blends. Again, consumers beware of mimickers. I like to refer to the Young Living oils as "GTG" (Genuine Therapeutic Grade)!

Obviously, if you can find the same standard of edible and impeccable clean, environmental sustainable essential oils then by all means, go ahead, they will be a great asset to you. There are some small and few companies that do . . . Make certain that they uphold to this high standard and you, the consumer, are wise to know a number of factors that make that difference, such as: the dedication of the grower; the location of where the plants are grown, method of farming, use of correct species, proper harvesting methods and the skill in distilling the oils, to name a few (much more is described in chapter 6).

Otherwise you will purchase essential oils that will not offer you all the marvellous benefits for skin care outlined in this guidebook. After all, the essential oil quality as nature provided is everything in achieving the desired results of health and glowing, radiant skin.

So I warn the reader once again: Buyer Beware! Quality products will not be found at department stores, discount stores, drug stores and beauty salons as they rarely contain pure essential oils. Many consumers are unaware that many health food store products or other direct selling essential oil companies contain adulterated oils (oils that have been processed with solvents/chemicals or have fillers/volumizers in them). The suggestions made throughout this guidebook apply to the use of Genuine, authentic and non-adulterated; 'therapeutic' grade A Essential Oils. I know that I am stressing this fact of 'purity' due to the potential 'risk' factor to you the buyer.

The company that I prefer to use and suggest to others—Young Living Company—encourages its Members or customers to visit the company's own and partnered biodynamic herbal or tree farms anywhere in the world. This allows you to become "in-touch" with and become "touched-by" the plants and the land. It was the greatest pleasure for me to meet D. Gary Young, president and founder of Young Living with his wife Mary Young. It was even more rewarding to travel with the Young's while on expeditions in visiting six of the global biodynamic herb farms. On numerous occasions, I witnessed the farming process from the planting of the seeds to the final product with D. Gary Young who gave thorough and detailed explanations. Hence the company has coined the phrase 'Seed to Seal' in claiming their distinction in the world's production of essential oils.

Today, I consider both Gary and Mary as my dear friends and Kindred Spirits. I have marveled at D. Gary Young's honoring and connectedness to commune with the Nature Spirits (in the plants, the animals, the trees) before planting and cutting the trees. Young Living's commitment to produce the finest and highest quality essential oils is unmatched in the world today. D. Gary Young is sought after for his knowledge and standards by many global markets.

Aromatherapy in ancient times was used for healing, beauty and medicine and considered a most precious substance that was the basis for trade for hundreds of years as evidenced with the Frankincense Trail documentation. You can become empowered and also enjoy the miracles that the botanicals offer on so many levels: mental, emotional and spiritual.

Now go to the mirror and see for yourself, who is staring back at you! Are you impressed? Do you have some mind-chatter going on in what you see? Are you pleased with the way you look? Well, the best motivation for change may be in what you see in the mirror.

I sincerely trust that this guidebook will inspire you to use herbal foods and essential oils, to continue your search and to further seek the treasures that are given to you from the sweet "nectar" of the plants. In Greek and Roman mythology, the drink of the gods was called 'nectar'—the drink that sustained their beauty and immortality. May you be blessed and enriched by the "essences" of the plants.

AND

"May your heart's garden of awakening bloom with a hundred flowers."
THICH NHAT HANH

POEM TO AN EGYPTIAN PRINCESS

She looks like the rising morning star,

At the start of a happy year,

Shining bright, fair of skin,

Lovely the look of her eyes,

Sweet the speech of her lips . . .

With graceful step she treads the ground,

Captures my heart by her movements,

She causes all men's necks to turn to see her,

Joy has he whom she embraces,

He is like the first of men!

Composed in Egypt between B.C. 1400 and 1200

which includes the reign of Akhenaton and Nefertiti B.C. 1375–1358

ACKNOWLEDGMENTS

I fully express my heartfelt appreciation to my family, to both my parents, mom and dad, who deeply instilled and impacted my life's ambitions and passions. I thank you dad for your determination, love and focus that has also been instrumental throughout my life. In your short time on this earth plane, you showed me much in being inventive and creative. I thank you dad and bless you in your afterlife journey. I love you dearly.

I especially thank you mom for supporting my enthusiasm and goals to be the best of who I can be. I honor your words of belief in me when I first began to write the 1st edition of this book in 2003. I am so appreciative of the love that you shared with me and your love that you poured out to all of your children. You were a beautiful woman not only in physical looks but with your heart and soul. I'm proud to embody the 'goodness', the 'kindness', and the inner beauty that you showed me throughout your life. Thank you for being my guide in teaching me the true essence of beauty, inside and out. I eternally give thanks and bless you in your spiritual journey. I love you dearly.

I thank my loving husband who patiently witnessed my long hours in preparing my first book and now my third edition amongst my many other authored books. You too supported my ideas and my vision in being of service to others, especially to making a positive difference in women's lives. It wasn't always easy for you when I would be so enraptured with my writing. I appreciate and love you for standing by.

I thank my loving family, my brothers, sister and sister-in-laws for their support and encouragement to continue with my many pursuits. They have always been available to help with family gatherings. I love you all. I specifically thank my younger brother Sal, for his encouraging words of being 'ahead of my time'. Thank You in following too in 'scents-a-tizing' your life and impacting the many around you in a positive, healthy way.

I also thank my many friends (too many to mention all of you and you know who you are) and other 'oilers' whom I have met over the years who encouraged and inspired me as well. I am grateful to all of you for your love, your light and your support of my ideas with my first edition that has now grown to its 3rd publication.

My deepest thanks go to D. Gary Young, founder/owner of Young Living Company who led the way for all of us. Gary, you made it all possible for me and the world to enjoy the essential oil treasures as we do. Your extraordinary gifts, dedication, your brilliance and your tireless giving to humanity has deeply shaped and blessed my life. I'm proud to be a partner with you in changing lives. Thank you for your love and the countless ways that you can make your visions a reality. Thank you for being such a far-sighted seer, a loving role model of hope and inspiration. No matter how big the challenges are that have come upon your path, you manage to find a creative way to victory. You are legendary in your insights, technology and bio-diverse farming practices. I love you wholeheartedly.

Most importantly, I am in full gratitude to God, our Divine Creator, the Infinite, for my inspiration, motivation, energy, life, beauty and courage. I also give thanks for the blessings that Creator has fashioned out of Mother Nature's precious plants that offer us their 'spirits', their treasured perfumery or aromas, their sacred essences—the essential oils for humanity.

I also thank a dear and loving friend, Anna-Maya Powell for her contribution to my first edition book. I thank and love you for your love, appreciation and encouragement over the years.

I give thanks to the many authors, researchers, teachers and models from whom I have learned. I thank all my students and clients who have embraced this work into their lives and have supported me in my continual search for truth, beauty, wellness and freedom.

Purposely kept to the last, I give a special acknowledgment to Mary Young who has written my foreword and for her on-going encouragement to me to expand my business pursuits and to continue to write and teach much of the research and information that is now contained in this 3rd edition book. I thank you Mary, for your insights, wisdom and love. Thank you for being my friend and a model to me and others in your inner and outer beauty. I love and appreciate you, dearly.

Lastly, I thank you, the reader for purchasing **Saving Face**. I trust that you will find many 'gems' to enhance your life. May you embody and express the fullness of your Divinity and your Feminine Beauty in its true exquisiteness and form.

In gratitude,

Sabina Mary DeVita

INTRODUCTION

LOOKING GOOD COULD BE KILLING YOU!

"One starts to get young at the age of sixty."
PABLO PICASSO

Pablo Picasso's statement above seems to hold a philosophy that shows great promise today for those seeking the true fountain of youth. Ever since the legend of the 16th century Spanish explorer Juan Ponce de León who was obsessed with the Fountain of Youth, the search for it still seems very much alive. Leon's obsession in finding the magical water source supposedly capable of reversing the aging process and curing sickness didn't happen but his travels did lead him to discover Florida, but not the fountain of youth.

The search for eternal youth, beauty and wellness has been with humankind for ages and is still a driving force today. It has resulted in a billion dollar industry!

There seems to be an insatiable thirst or hunger for immortality, youthfulness and /or aging gracefully. In order to unlock the secrets to the aging phenomenon, we need to understand the many areas that impact us in the 'aging' process from a philosophical point of view as well as to the spiritual/mental/emotional and physical aspects.

No one wants or likes to hear their doctor say "your condition is due to your age" or "What do you expect at your age?" I certainly didn't either. What I did know when I started this path to greater ways in aging or in getting older was simply this—I could choose differently from my parents. My father passed away when he was only 63—being a heavy smoker early in his life, it took his life force all too early. When I witnessed the amount of drugs, surgeries and injuries that my mother experienced in her lifetime, I saw how she suffered more pain and ailments later on as she aged. When I became more involved with natural, holistic health, I was able to help my mom and I believe, help her to live longer into her 80s with fewer to no drugs.

Can we change the paradigm of aging? I believe we need to philosophically redefine aging. What are the held and taught beliefs within our society about aging? How are the cultural held view-points impacting you, me and everyone? What does the 'retirement age' mean? What does the statement "I am retired" create psychologically and in the body?

What happens when you consider yourself as: 'over the hill', 'time to retire', 'getting old' or 'having a senior moment', or anything else that is robbing you of the possibility of you generating your life and your body in a different, youthful way? What is your viewpoint about yourself? What is your belief about aging? How do you speak about yourself in getting older?

The new 'quantum physics' world view has been showing us that we, as energy systems create ourselves from moment to moment. We create our own realities—our thoughts, our emotions do in fact paint our world, create our world. Dr. Christiane Northrup in her video presentation on aging, emphatically points out that as a culture; we're programmed to dread an inevitable decline in all facets of our lives as we age. That is how society and most world cultures define aging. Yet this belief is distorted and certainly excludes the new discoveries in quantum science and who we are. The dictum is simply this: we do create our reality and we can change for a better, longer, healthier life by understanding the power of our minds.

The influence of the mind, intention and the power of visualization with emotions can empower us if we know how to use them. How do you visualize yourself . . . what would you like to look like and feel like?—take a moment now as you are reading this book. What is your vision of you as you progress in years? How do you picture or consider yourself now? What will you be doing in 10 years, 20 years or 50 years time from now? How will you look and feel? Begin now to make the changes that will support the quality of your life for the better and for your future. It starts with your thoughts—your imagination, your beliefs and your action. It truly is an inside-out not from outside-in process!

Albert Einstein understood the importance of the creative mind when he stated: "Imagination is more important than knowledge, for while knowledge points to all there is, imagination points to all there will be."

Suzanne Somers, author of **Bombshell** writes about how she illustrated the power of her 'imagination' while experiencing radiation treatments in the hospital for her breast cancer. She came to realize that she had the ultimate choice to make between—her sickness, feeling sorry for herself or true health and wellness. She decided to fully commit to a natural wellness lifestyle and came to terms with her adversities. Her pivotal decision was: to see herself healthy, to visualize a different end-point. When she made 'that' decision for a better life she took control of her destiny. She has now become a pillar of light and hope for thousands of others and not just in the alternative health field. I applaud her victories and her tremendous accomplishments not only as an actress, but as a best-selling author and caring, forward thinking human being.

Professor Emeritus William A. Tiller, of Stanford University's Department of Materials Science, has for over 30 years, been pursuing serious experimental and theoretical study of the field of psychoenergetics. His pursuit of the power of human intention over the physical world has proven that indeed intention does in fact affect our physical reality!

What happens by holding to an old belief? Redefine Aging in a quantum world.

Records show that Biblical figures like Moses lived a long life of hundreds of years. The quest to achieve such longevity has certainly become more mainstream. Anti-aging and retaining one's beauty, in fact, has developed into a booming 20th century industry. Glamour magazines, the media, have created an image for both men and women as to what they should look like and how to feel. Anti-aging products have become so popularized, (the fastest growing sector of the cosmetic industry)—so much so that it has developed into a dangerously toxic and costly way of life. Women and men are becoming rapidly more obsessed with looking and feeling young and beautiful with the fake promises of the advertising campaigns. It doesn't have to be. The industry has addressed the issues superficially—truly missing the meaning of what I would consider 'Beauty' to be—one that comes from an inner state, a healthy toxic-free body, and a consciousness of grace, love, inner peace and happiness.

But in order to understand what is happening in the beauty field, let's look at some of these outrageous statistics.

- $500 billion is normally spent each year for chemical beauty aids & beauty treatments of all types in the United States and Canada.
- Many billions are being spent for preparations containing harmful, irritating and dangerous poisons but not only that . . .
- Almost 15 million plastic surgery procedures were performed around the world in 2011, according to a study by the International Society for Aesthetic Plastic Surgeons (ISAPS) & more than 21% of those took place in the US.
- In 2013, the numbers increased substantially: More than 23 million cosmetic surgical and nonsurgical procedures were performed worldwide
- ISAPS reports that their latest 2014 statistics indicate that cosmetic surgery is on the rise on a global scale. Rankings are based solely on those countries

from which a sufficient survey response was received and data were considered to be representative.

- Botox injections (botulism bacteria—the most severe type of food poisoning) came out on top as the most popular procedure, with over 3 million injections of botulinum toxin (type A) having been administered worldwide back in 2011 (reported in U.S. news blog).
- ISAPS reports that the leading nonsurgical procedures performed in 2013 were:
  - Botulinum Toxin (5,145,189)
  - Fillers and Resorbables (3,089,686)
  - Laser Hair Removal (1,440,252)
  - Non-Invasive Facial Rejuvenation (1,307,300)
  - Chemical Peel, CO2 resurfacing, dermabrasion (773,442)
  - Botox is the Second-most popular prescription drug in the world!
    Dr. Oz reports an increase of 600% Botox injections over the last 10 years . . . and it's not only for women, men are just as intrigued.

WHY IS BOTOX DANGEROUS?

(Besides causing paralysis and even death—see section: *The Anti-Aging Boom: what is the cost?*)

- According to a May 19, 2013 ABC News article it highlights the recent increase in the popularity of Botox for those under the age of thirty—many in their 20s!
- Patients who have not reached thirty are having Botox injections . . . to look fresh and beautiful as long as possible—calling it a proactive measure!
- According to a study published in the Journal of Neuroscience, 2009 and reported by Natural News: The botulinum toxin injected into the face from the popular drug Botox can move into the brain, where it may cause damage to the central nervous system.

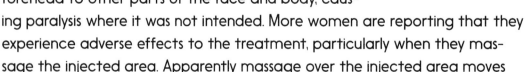

- More and more reports are showing that Botox isn't as safe as it seems. The toxin can spread from the forehead to other parts of the face and body, causing paralysis where it was not intended. More women are reporting that they experience adverse effects to the treatment, particularly when they massage the injected area. Apparently massage over the injected area moves the toxin around the body and can cause headaches and other side effects such as droopy eyelids and more (Natural News).

- Black Market Botox: is also on the rise and Hurting People. People in many cities in the U.S. have been busted for injecting Botox without a license. Home parties offering inexpensive Botox injections has become more common-place.
- Even doctors have been duped by buying less expensive (most often black-market tainted Botox) on-line causing serious reactions to those that receive these injections.
- WOW!—What are women and men doing for the sake of beauty and youthfulness?
- And with a society so focused on looking the part—even children and teenagers are being subjected to Botox and surgery: The number of teens and children getting plastic surgery has gone up 30 percent over the last decade, with more young people resorting to operations in order to avoid bullying or to fit in. (Huffington Post)

Ponce's quest certainly rages on but it still isn't the promised land of the fountain of youth.

MEN TOO

The business of grooming and looking younger for Men is booming. Men are spending more on skin care services and products than ever before.

The 2010 American Society of Plastic Surgeons (ASPS) statistics show that men underwent more than 1.1 million cosmetic procedures, both minimally-invasive and surgical. But for 2013, ISAPS reports that Men had more than 3 million cosmetic procedures; 12.8% of the total.

- The majority of the top 10 fastest-growing cosmetic procedures for men were surgical in contrast to the previous explosive growth in minimally-invasive treatments.
- Every day more and more men are undergoing cosmetic surgery procedures to correct signs of aging, improve their appearance and keep their bodies in sync with their youthful souls—as advertised in 2014 by one Cosmetic surgery institute in Toronto, Ontario Canada.
- Some of the procedures include:
  - Botox—to remove the tired, angry look. Erase frown lines and stop under-arm sweating
  - Fillers—to fill in deep creases and to add volume to an aging face

— Non-Surgical Facelift procedures use a combination of Botox and fillers such as Voluma or Perlane to help to lift the face in a non-surgical manner

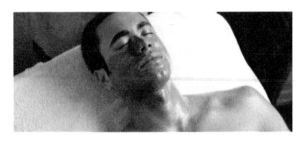

According to a 2012 Mintel research study, men are spending more cash on skin care services at salons. They point out that 52% of men have used professional care services. 25% of Men in the 18–34 year old category report having a manicure or pedicure. Also, 38% of men in the 18 to 34-year-old category have had a facial or body treatment, compared to only 15% of men 55 and up. Research also reveals that 20% of men and 22% of women in the same age range have had a facial at a salon. Mintel research says there is a growing trend among the male population to look clean and groomed.

The search for the Fountain of Youth continues in another arena, not for Ponce's magical water source but in the laboratory, as one research team discovered, what they call: the new Fountain of youth 'gene'.

Experts have long been puzzled as to why young animals recover from injuries more quickly than adults and were able to isolate the gene. The gene, Lin28a, is highly active in unborn children, in the embryonic development but does less and less with age. Harvard researchers now hope that waking the gene up in adults could speed healing of wounds after operations. As published in the journal **Cell**, the researchers say that it may also be possible to create a drug that works in the same way.

In a culture that puts a premium on youth, it's easy to see why we're always looking for anti-aging remedies, even the new so-called anti-aging drugs. But the era of main stage pharmaceuticals is coming to a crisis as well since more awakened individuals are recognizing the harmful, toxic side effects to themselves and the environment with the synthetic drug world.

We are witnessing the environmental devastations and the demise of our young and old who succumb to the 'drug dictates'. Adding to our debilitation and in many cases the cause of our illnesses, is the use of these toxic, often times dangerous, cosmetic, personal and home care products, unbeknownst and unknown to the average consumer. Many of the harmful toxic effects will be outlined in the next few chapters in order to understand why we need to stop them. I have also presented the latest statistics of major diseases with dementia and Alzheimer's leading the way. What are we thinking or perhaps we are not, in what we are doing to ourselves and our planet?

Suzanne Somers states it well: "In fact, the overuse of drugs for every ailment is robbing our brains, leading us right to our final rest stop, the nursing homes, where patients require more and more drugs to facilitate every function of their bodies" (**Bombshell:** page 14). I like to add to this statement that the 'toxic chemical soup overuse' from our everyday living products like hairsprays to soap, to laundry detergents to lipstick, to hand sanitizers are not only robbing our brains but blocking our brains and disconnecting us from our Infinite Higher Source (Vibrational Cleaning.com)!

Some of the Baby boomers along with our younger generation are waking up to understanding the long-term side effects of taking so many toxic drugs, the overuse of the chemicals in our homes, our cosmetics, the poisoning of our lands from the pesticides, insecticides, herbicides absorbed into our GMO foods and our poisoned fluoridated, chlorinated and polluted water. There are many more yet to awaken to this 'toxic' world.

The goal of this book as with my **Vibrational Cleaning** books is to enlighten the masses even more, so the 'enlightened minority' can become the enlightened, conscientious majority. The rest of this chapter and chapter 1 describe the dangers of our cosmetic industry, an unregulated, sinister industry that is all about profits!

More notable conscientious scientists are also becoming aware of the demands for more chemical-free, or ECO friendly or Eco-Green products. These scientists from prestigious universities are presently researching and discovering nutraceuticals and stem cell uses for the real, true 'fountain of youth'.

The challenge for us is simply this: what is true and what is hype? What is real green and what is Greenwashing? I present some of the anti-aging research and supplement uses in Chapter 7 and in Chapters 8 to 9, I outline the many benefits of 100% genuine essential oil protocols that can be used directly on the face and the body.

"Cancer and health risk experts just concluded reviews that indicate mainstream cosmetics and personal hygiene products pose the highest cancer risk exposures to the general public, higher than smoking."

Cancer Prevention Coalition
press release, June 17, 2002

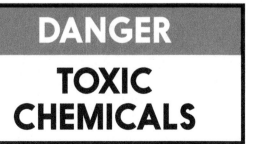

CHAPTER 1

COSMETICS ARE FOR PROFIT–NOT FOR PEOPLE

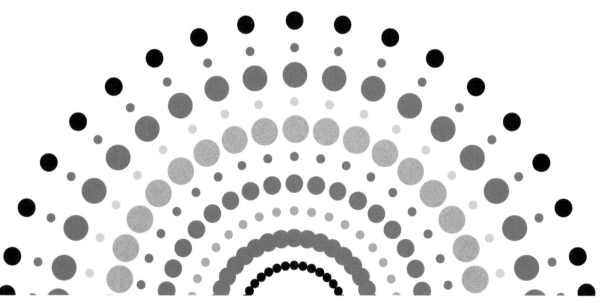

"The FDA can take action on a case in which harm is done only after a product is on the market and only after it has received enough consumer complaints and enough evidence has been collected to prove in court that the product is hazardous."
DEBRA LYNN DADD

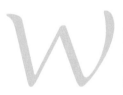hat is engine degreaser doing on your face? Or how about antifreeze under your armpits and on your lips? Sounds ridiculous, I know. But keep using these personal care items and you'll need a side order of ***Chemo!***

In other words, when you start to investigate the ingredients in cosmetics and personal care items, it's quite loud and clear that the chemicals are Carcinogenic! **Simply put, they are cancer causing.** Sadly, most products are made from petrochemical derivatives of non-renewable crude oil (not found in nature) that cause cancer, are neurotoxins and can even act as mutagens which means they can change the genetic coding in your cells. Mineral oil for example, is widely used in lotions, cosmetics and other mineral-oil based products that are toxic to the human body. It is the same substance that kills marine life after an oil spill in the ocean. When the oils are hydrogenated, basically making them act like plastic—the human body doesn't know what to do with it. All kinds of side effects can occur—such as fatigue, memory loss, personality changes, headaches, sleep disturbances and sexual dysfunction as well as causing cancer.

What I also find appalling is the number of lubricants, cosmetics, waxes and soaps that are made from animal renderings. The remains of slaughtered, diseased and euthanized animals are dumped into huge grinders, mixed together and steam-cooked. The fatty substance that floats to the top is used to make a fatty substance used in your common household products! Now how appetizing and healthy is that (Mad Cowboy Reference)?

The number 1 health problem in the world today is due in great part to the toxic chemical exposures. All diseases will have some association with toxic chemicals. No one escapes it.

The organization 'Safer Chemicals, Healthy Families' released a report called "**The Health Case for Reforming the Toxic Substances Control Act.**" to raise awareness of the most dangerous chemicals in order to help reform the current laws in the U.S.

According to their report, 133 million people in the USA—almost half of all Americans—are now living with chronic diseases and conditions related to toxic chemical exposures, which now account for 70% of deaths and 75% of US health care costs. They calculate that if only a fraction of toxic chemicals were removed from consumer products, it would save the U.S. health care system an estimated $5 billion every year. (Safer Chemicals, Healthy Families)

It is actually quite shocking that these toxins are still allowed with the escalating numbers in cancer alone! Dr. Samuel Epstein, chairman of the Cancer Prevention Coalition and emeritus Professor of Occupational and Environmental Medicine at the University of Illinois, School of Public Health at Chicago and leading international authority on "toxicology" and the carcinogenic effects of contaminants in consumer products, warns women of the harmful chemicals that may cause an **unreasonable cancer risk** to them.

He points out that it is "unthinkable that women would knowingly inflict such exposures on their infants and children and themselves if the products routinely used were labeled with explicit warnings of cancer risks."

It is also unbelievable that the powerful multi-billion-dollar global industries continue to inflict such risks on the unsuspecting consumers, especially when safe alternatives are available.

Dr. Epstein has authored 270 scientific articles and 15 books on the causes and prevention of cancer. These include the groundbreaking: *The Politics of Cancer Revisited and Unreasonable Risk* (1979), *The Safe Shopper's Bible, Breast Cancer Prevention Program* and most recently *Toxic Beauty* (2009) about carcinogens and other toxic ingredients in cosmetics and personal care products. Dr. Epstein's latest book, (2010) is called *Healthy Beauty*.

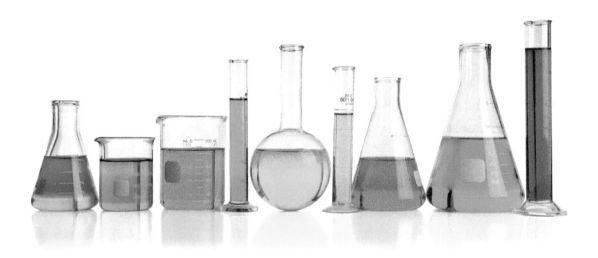

The whole cosmetic industry is a totally unregulated industry, taking the position of "innocent until proven guilty" to the use of any ingredients. Even the use of the word natural can be used by anyone.

... almost half of all Americans—are now living with chronic diseases and conditions related to toxic chemical exposures

Unless a chemical used in the beauty and personal care product is proven to cause harm to human health, it is classified as GRAS, or "generally recognized as safe." In **Unreasonable Risk,** Epstein points out how the alarming cancer statistics has escalated to endemic proportions in industrialized nations worldwide.

In the United States alone, risks of cancer are one in two for men and one in three for women. Since the 1940s, the incidence of non-smoking cancers in the U.S. during the 1990s increased approximately as follows:

TYPES OF CANCERS

- Prostate cancer, non-Hodgkin's lymphoma, multiple myeloma—200%
- Thyroid cancer—155%
- Testicular cancer—120%
- Adult brain and nervous system cancer—70%
- Female breast cancer—60%
- Childhood cancer—35%

As posted on Dr. Epstein's site: since passage of the 1971 National Cancer Act, the overall incidence of cancer in the U.S. has escalated to epidemic magnitude, now striking 1.3 million and killing about 550,000 annually. The median age for the diagnosis of cancer is 67 in adults and six in children.

According to the States Medical and Scientific Adviser, World Cancer Research Fund International, they report high international numbers. *"There were an estimated 14.1 million cancer cases around the world in 2012. The number is expected to rise to 19.3 million by 2025."*

Cancer Rates in Japan have been sharply increasing as well, e.g. 100% increase in multiple myeloma in both sexes; 80% increase in ovarian cancer and 300% increase in lymphatic leukemia.

Dr. Epstein continues to state that while the cancer risks have escalated, the "cure" for cancers has remained relatively unchanged for decades. The predominant cause, Dr. Epstein states "is based on a strong body of scientific evidence incriminating the role of run-away technologies, particularly the petrochemical and nuclear industries."

He continues to state that cancer is mainly caused by chemical and physical agents in the environment. Our total environment and the public at large are unknowingly exposed to avoidable carcinogens in food, household cleaners and products, cosmetics, prescription drugs and toiletries.

> . . . cancer is mainly caused by chemical and physical agents in the environment. Our total environment and the public at large are unknowingly exposed to avoidable carcinogens in food, household cleaners and products, cosmetics, prescription drugs and toiletries.

Clearly, the general public are not being warned of these avoidable carcinogens. Why? According to Epstein, a major part is due to the fact that the National Cancer Institute (NCI) has no interest whatsoever in prevention. Its focus is exclusively focused on diagnosed treatment and oncology research.

The NCI has failed to develop or publicize any listing or registry to avoid all exposures to carcinogens.

Furthermore Dr. Epstein states, *NCI (National Cancer Institute) has failed to respond, except misleadingly, to a series of congressional requests for such information ... In March, 1988, in a series of questions to NCI director Richard Klausner . . . "We requested information on NCI's policies and priorities, and Congressman Obey said, "Should the NCI develop or register avoidable carcinogens and to make this information widely available to the public?" and the answer was, and remains, "No."*

It is well known that the pharmaceutical companies largely control the FDA and that they financially fund the elected officials. This obviously creates a conflict of interest.

To give you, the reader, an example of the extent of the carcinogenic exposures found in our cosmetics, a sample of one product from the, **The Politics of Cancer Revisited** book is given on the following page.

Cover Girl Replenishing Natural Finish Make-Up (Foundation)
PROCTER & GAMBLE, INC. LABELED TOXIC INGREDIENTS

- **BHA**, carcinogenic; TALC, carcinogenic;

- **TITANIUM DIOXIDE**, carcinogenic;

- **TRIETHANOLAMINE (TEA)**, interacts with nitrites to form carcinogenic nitrosamines;

- **LANOLIN**, often contaminated with DDT and other carcinogenic pesticides.

- **PARABENS**, Contact dermatitis.

- **FRAGRANCE**, Wide range of unlabeled, untested, and toxic ingredients; contact dermatitis.

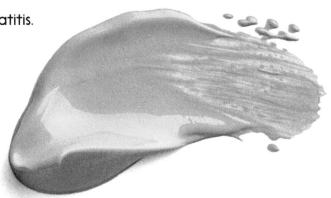

(Epstein, 1998, page 480)

Dr. Epstein also has serious concerns about cosmetic products containing **nano-particles**. These nano-particles are being used in many different brands of cosmetics and **cosmeceuticals** and that the facts about these technologies are being hidden and ignored. In his 2010 interview with Dr. Mercola, he specifically points out that **nano-particles** are the **most serious, known dangerous substance in cosmetic use worldwide.**

Dr. Epstein refers to these nano-particles as "universal asbestos." He warns that: *"There is no labeling of the warning at all of the dangers of these nanoparticles, instead they are touted as reducing wrinkling and firming up the skin surface," "However, the use of nanoparticles in cosmeceuticals (mainly used in cosmeceuticals) whether they are sham cosmeceuticals or whether they're bonafide cosmeceuticals, poses an extraordinarily dangerous and unrecognized public health hazard.*

"Nanoparticles, because of their ultramicroscopic size, readily penetrate the skin, can invade underlying blood vessels, get into the general blood stream, and produce distant toxic effects. We already have evidence of this, including toxic effects in the brain, degenerative disorders in the brain, and nerve damage. So we're dealing here with one of the most dangerous types of products in the whole cosmetic industry."

Epstein continues to state with great passion that nanoparticles should be banned. He also points out that in mid-2008, *"The British Royal Commission report warned that products that contain nanoparticles pose very, very high toxic risks."*

Epstein continues to add: *". . . the evidence which we've accumulated so far, is largely restricted to the fact that they [nano particles] get into your bloodstream and reach organs throughout your body. And as far as the brain is concerned, we have actual evidence of entry into the brain and producing toxic effects—lesions, small lesions, toxic effects in the brain."*

Dr. Stephen and Gina Antczak in **Cosmetics Unmasked** point out how contaminated cosmetics and toiletries are more common than what we would like to believe.

Some of these harmful ingredients are presented in this chapter for this purpose to raise awareness of these dangers in an unregulated industry. I then provide a "Scents-able," simple, way to create your own solution to Natural Green Beauty and how to wipe years off your face—wisely and safely in the later chapters!

The National Institute of Occupational Safety and Health administration (OSHA) has identified **884 toxic** or potentially cancer causing agents used in everyday personal care products. They identified 778 to cause acute toxic effects:

- 146 cause tumors (some that are cancerous)
- 314 cause developmental abnormalities (adversely affecting the fetus during pregnancies)
- 376 can cause skin and eye damage
- 218 cause reproductive problems

The FDA has committed no resources for assessing chemical safety.

Dr. Epstein has classified chemical ingredients as ones that directly cause cancer and those that are hidden (causing cancer under certain conditions). There are over 40 carcinogens used in mainstream industry such as **BHT/BHA, coal tar dyes, FD & C colors, fluoride, formaldehyde, saccharin, talc, titanium dioxide, and (DEA) diethanolamine and over 30 that are hidden such as sodium lauryl sulfate, aflatoxin, arsenic, crystalline silica, organochlorine pesticides in lanolin** to name a few including:

- Ethylene oxide
- 1–4 Dioxane
- Nitrosamines
- Acrylamide
- For example, 1–4 dioxane, a by-product of the cancer-causing petrochemical Ethylene Oxide are both well-known carcinogens. Ethylene oxide is listed

by the `Campaign for Safe Cosmetics` as a known human carcinogen. A March 14, 2008 study commissioned by the Organic Consumers Association (OCA) found that many leading "natural" and "organic" brand shampoos, body washes and lotions contain the carcinogenic contaminant 1,4-Dioxane. Sadly, Companies that donate to breast cancer research still use carcinogens in their products!

- The California EPA listed 1,4-Dioxane—as a kidney toxicant, neurotoxicant and respiratory toxi-cant, among others.

- It is also a leading groundwater contaminant. It is hidden in ingredients such as PEG, polysorbates, laureth, ethoxylated alcohols.

- It is also very commonly used in personal care products and in cosmetics that are easily absorbed through the skin.

- Its carcinogenicity was first reported in 1965, and later confirmed in studies including one from the National Cancer Institute in 1978.

- Much more of the toxicity of these chemicals are discussed in the book, **Vibrational Cleaning.**

The numbers of chemicals in our products are staggering and too many to mention them all in this guidebook. Some of the main ones have been highlighted for you. For the most part, if you can't read it or pronounce its name, then it is most likely a chemical to avoid. Here are a few of the main ones to be aware of as described below.

DIETHANOLAMINE (DEA) OR TRIETHANOLAMINE (TEA)

One of the most common ingredients and a toxic compound found in personal care products is **diethanolamine (DEA)** or **triethanolamine (TEA)** used by metal workers as surfactant or detergent. It reacts with nitrite preservatives (found in cosmetics or toiletries and also in preserved meats such as cold cuts, bacon and ham) to form a potent carcinogen **nitrosodiethanolamine (NDELA)**, well recognized by federal agencies and institutions and the World Health Organization.

DEA was found to induce liver and kidney cancer. Dr. Epstein has issued stern warnings regarding the use of cocamide DEA or Lauramide DEA.

DEA is used in shampoos, hair conditioners, cleansers, cosmetics and lotions, was found in over 600 home and personal care products.

DEA is not excreted easily from the body and accumulates in the fatty tissues of the brain, liver, kidneys and spleen with repeated exposures. This leads to mounting tissue and nerve damage. In 1979, the FDA published a notice to the cosmetic industry to immediately remove the carcinogen DEA/TEA from cosmetics. In spite of this, DEA is still one of the most commonly used ingredients in personal care products. (27 out of 29 products surveyed in 1991 found concentrations of this carcinogen, which was confirmed by the FDA). Unfortunately, mainstream U.S. industry has been unresponsive and *even to the extent of ignoring an explicit warning by the Cosmetics, Toiletries and Fragrance Association to discontinue uses of DEA"* (Epstein, 1998). It is a reckless decision on the part of the industry. You the consumer are being made aware of this so you can make safe and wise choices in purchasing your products. Consumer power is in your pocket book.

According to Dr. Antczak, the three most notorious contaminants are **1, 4-dioxane, nitrosamines and endocrine disrupter chemicals** or "gender benders" (more in Chapter 4). They also point out that 1,4-dioxane is carcinogenic and readily penetrates human skin.

Dr. Hulda Clark, author of **A Cure For All Advanced Cancers**, issued a stern warning about another chemical called **propyl alcohol**, an antiseptic commonly used in cosmetics (another toxic compound) found in shampoos, rubbing alcohol, mouthwash, all shaving supplies, including **all bottled water, white sugar**, carbonated beverages and decaffeinated coffee. She claims that this is the basis for causing many cancers. This may seem radical, but she advises do protect yourself.

TRICLOSAN

Triclosan is another very common and toxic chemical found in too many of our products. It is a pesticide, an antimicrobial chemical, most commonly used in hand soaps and body washes to inhibit bacterial growth. Triclosan is also used as an antibacterial agent in laundry detergent, facial tissues, toothpaste, clothing and antiseptics for wounds, as well as a preservative to resist bacteria, fungus, mildew and odors in other household products that are sometimes advertized as "anti-bacterial". These products include garbage bags, toys, linens, mattresses, toilet fixtures, computer keyboards, clothing, furniture fabric and paints. Triclosan also has medical applications.

Triclosan is absorbed through the skin and has been detected in human breast milk, blood and urine samples. It has been linked to hormone disruption in laboratory studies. The chemical does not degrade easily and is toxic to aquatic wildlife. It is implicated in the rise of the 'Superbug' or the flesh-eating disease.

Most recently in 2014, the *Environmental Science and Technology Journal* published a study on the human "Fetal Exposure to Triclosan and Triclocarban in an Urban Population" from Brooklyn, New York.

The researchers found that all 181 urine samples contained high levels of antibacterial ingredient triclosan and the chemical was present in just over half of all umbilical cord blood samples. The Food and Drug Administration, found no evidence that triclosan in antibacterial soaps provide any benefit over washing with regular soap and water, yet many companies continue to add it to their consumer products.

U.S. researchers report that **one in eight of the 82,000 ingredients** used in personal care products are industrial chemicals, including carcinogens, pesticides, reproductive toxins, and hormone disruptors. Many products include plasticizers (chemicals that keep concrete soft), degreasers (used to get grime off auto parts), and surfactants (they reduce surface tension in water, like in paint and inks). (Environmental Working Group ewg. org) You can well imagine what that does to your skin, to your organs, nerves and brain as well as to the environment!

Now that is not all . . . **Heavy metal exposure** is more common than we realize in cosmetics as well. Acute heavy metal toxicity like lead, aluminum, copper, uranium and mercury, has been a concern in the workplace or from an occupational accident for years. But it is being used in common everyday products causing chronic heavy metal toxicity build-up in the system—it remains a silent killer.

Many of the cosmetic products sold in stores contain small trace elements of heavy metals.

Many of the cosmetic products sold in stores contain small trace elements of heavy metals. These metals act as free radicals in the body, (more on free radicals in chapter 4) damaging healthy cells and encouraging rapid cell death which simply means it is accelerating aging. Your anti-aging serum could be aging you sooner than helping you.

A 2014 study by the Centre for Science and Environment's Pollution Monitoring Lab found measurable levels of **mercury in 44% of skin creams, along with chromium and nickel in about 50% of lipsticks tested.**

- Another new analysis of lead in lipstick conducted by the U.S. Food and Drug Administration in 2014 reveals that the problem of lead in lipstick is worse and more widespread than previously reported.
- The new study **found lead in 400 lipsticks tested** by the agency, at widely varying levels of up to 7.19 parts per million (ppm)—**more than twice the levels reported** in a previous FDA study.

As outlined earlier, there are no laws requiring cosmetic manufacturers to label their products. According to a 2004 study by the Environmental Working Group, the number of toxic metals found in blood samples from new born babies is on average 287, which includes mercury, fire retardants, pesticides and chemicals from non stick cook ware (articles.mercola.com, 2015).

LEST WE FORGET: COGNITIVE DECLINE

The links of these toxic chemicals to other diseases are also devastatingly on the rise in **Alzheimer's and Parkinson's**. Researchers are pointing out that the rise of cognitive decline is being linked to environmental chemicals and contaminants throughout one's lifespan. Extensive laboratory and epidemiologic evidence now shows that certain kinds of pesticide exposures increase the risk of Parkinson's.

Parkinson's 50,000 new cases diagnosed annually expected to double by 2030.

Alzheimer's 5.4 million in the U.S. (2/3 are women) expected to triple to 6 million by 2050.

www.saferchemicals.org/health-report

SUMMARY CHART
TOXIC OFFENDERS & THE GRAVE DIGGERS

INGREDIENT	USE	DANGERS
Triclosan	Used in antibacterial cosmetics, such as toothpastes, cleansers and antiperspirants. Used in cleaners, used as an antibacterial agent in laundry detergent, facial tissues, and antiseptics for wounds, as well as a preservative. These products include garbage bags, toys, linens, mattresses, toilet fixtures, clothing, furniture fabric, and paints. computer keyboards—over 1200 products Triclosan also has medical applications.	Interferes with hormone function (endocrine disrupter) and may contribute to antibiotic resistance in bacteria. Harmful to fish and other wildlife. Doesn't easily degrade and builds up in the environment as well as human tissue.
Mineral Oil, Paraffin, and Petrolatum	In hair products, lip balm, skin care products. A petroleum product, petrolatum can be contaminated with polycyclic aromatic hydrocarbons (PAHs). Studies suggest that exposure to PAHs—including skin contact over extended periods of time—is associated with cancer	These petroleum products coat the skin like plastic—clogs pores and creates a build-up of toxins Blocks all nutrients—no such thing as a good mineral oil! Can slow cellular development, creating earlier signs of aging. Can disrupt hormonal activity. The European Union classifies petrolatum a carcinogen ii and restricts its use in cosmetics. PAHs in petrolatum can also cause skin irritation and allergies Think about black oil pumped from deep underground and putting this on your skin!

INGREDIENT	USE	DANGERS
DEA-related ingredients Look also for related chemicals MEA and TEA	Used in creamy and foaming products, such as moisturizers and shampoos.	Can react to form nitrosamines, which may cause cancer. Harmful to fish and other wildlife. Causes mild to moderate skin and eye irritation. Higher doses known to cause liver cancers. The Danish Environmental Protection Agency classifies cocamide DEA as hazardous to the environment because of its acute toxicity to aquatic organisms and potential for bioaccumulation.
Dibutyl phthalate (DBP)	Used mainly in nail products as a solvent for dyes and as a plasticizer that prevents nail polishes from becoming brittle. Phthalates are also used as fragrance ingredients in many other cosmetics, but consumers won't find these listed on the label.	In laboratory experiments, it has been shown to cause developmental defects, changes in the testes and prostate, and reduced sperm counts. Health Canada notes evidence suggesting that exposure to phthalates may cause health effects such as liver and kidney failure in young children when products containing phthalates are sucked or chewed for extended periods.
Hydroquinone	Used for lightening skin.	Banned in the UK, rated most toxic on the EWG's Skin Deep database, and linked to cancer and reproductive toxicity.

INGREDIENT	USE	DANGERS
Lead	Used in lipsticks	Known carcinogen found in lipstick and hair dye, but never listed because it's a contaminant, not an ingredient.
Formaldehyde	Building materials, particle boards, plywood, and fiberboard; glues and adhesives; permanent-press fabrics; and many toiletries, hair care products, perfumes and any Fragrant product.	Causes cancer. Also causes coughing and wheezing. asthma, It is known as a "sensitizer," causes allergic reactions, itchy skin, rashes.
Placental extract:	Skin care cremes	Used in some skin and hair products, but linked to endocrine disruption.
Sodium laurel or lauryl sulfate (SLS), also known as sodium laureth sulfate (SLES)	Found in over 90% of personal care products!	SLS combined with other chemicals may become a "nitrosamine"—a potent carcinogen. SLS may damage the liver. It is harmful to aquatic and wild life breaks down your skin's moisture barrier, potentially leading to dry skin with premature aging. Due to its easy penetration on your skin, allows for easy access to other chemicals
Acrylamide	Found in many facial creams	Linked to mammary tumors
Propylene glycol	Common cosmetic moisturizer and carrier for fragrance oils.	Known to cause dermatitis and skin irritation. May inhibit skin cell growth. Linked to kidney and liver problems.
Phenol carbolic acid	Found in many lotions and skin creams.	Can cause circulatory collapse, paralysis, convulsions, coma, and even death from respiratory failure.

INGREDIENT	USE	DANGERS
Dioxane	Hidden in ingredients such as PEG, polysorbates, laureth, ethoxylated alcohols. Used heavily in laundry detergents. Very common in personal care products.	Usually contaminated with high concentrations of highly volatile 1,4-dioxane that's easily absorbed through the skin—it's highly carcinogenic. Nasal passages are considered extremely vulnerable.
Toluene	Is a very toxic chemical made from petroleum and coal tar . . . found in most synthetic fragrances and nail polish.	Chronic exposure linked to anemia, lowered blood cell count, liver or kidney damage . . . may affect a developing fetus.
BHA and BHT BHA (butylated hydroxyanisole) and BHT (butylated hydroxytoluene)	These are closely related synthetic antioxidants used as preservatives in lipsticks and moisturizers, make up, among other cosmetics. They are also widely used as food preservatives.	Suspected endocrine disruptors and may cause cancer (BHA). Harmful to fish and other wildlife.
Parabens	Heavily used preservatives in the cosmetic industry; and household cleaners, shampoos make-up - used in an estimated 13,200 cosmetic and skin care products.	Studies implicate their connection with cancer, especially associated with breast cancer. Mimics estrogen thus interferes with hormone-disruptive to your body's endocrine system.
Coal tar dyes: **p-phenylenediamine** and colours listed as "CI" followed by a five digit number	Coal tar-derived colours are used extensively in cosmetics and in hair dyes - especially darker hair dyes.	Coal tar is a mixture of many chemicals, derived from petroleum, Coal tar is recognized as a human carcinogen and the main concern with individual coal tar colours (whether produced from coal tar or synthetically) is their potential to cause cancer. Can be contaminated with heavy metals and aluminum-toxic to the brain.

Sources:
David Suzuki site http://davidsuzuki.org/issues/health/science/toxics/chemicals-in-your-cosmetics Environmental Working Group—Skin Deep Guide www.ewg.org
Safer chemicals health report http://saferchemicals.org/health-report.

CONSUMER BEWARE!

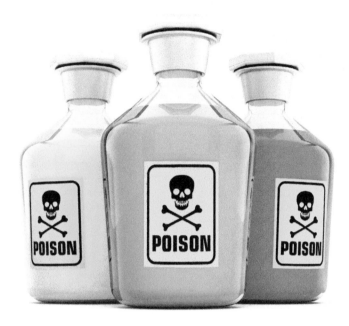

Even labels marked with "organic" are misleading. **Companies can say it's "made with organic" if it contains a minimum of 70 percent certified-organic ingredients. However, that still leaves 30 percent for toxins.**

'If you can't eat it then don't wear it on your skin.'

FACT:

Federal law allows companies to leave some chemical ingredients off their product labels, including those considered to be trade secrets, components of fragrance and nano-materials (FDA 2011). Fragrance may include any number of the industry's 3,100 stock chemicals (IFRA 2010), none of which is required to be listed on labels. Tests of fragrance ingredients have found an average of 14 hidden compounds per formulation, including ingredients linked to hormone disruption and sperm damage (EWG & CSC 2010).

CHAPTER 2

FRAGRANCES AND OTHER TOXINS

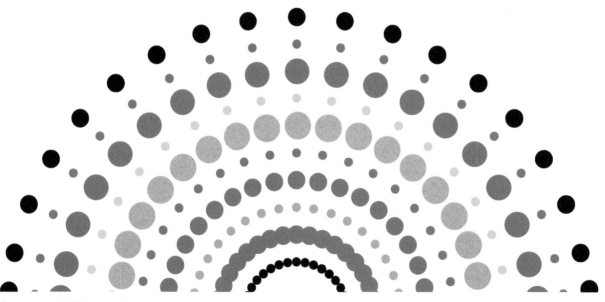

*"How old would you be if you
didn't know how old you are?"*
LEROY (SATCHEL) PAIGE

Fragrances also pose a serious health risk, often poorly recognized and an important source of indoor air pollution. There are more than 5,000 chemicals used in the manufacture of fragrances and according to a report from the National Institute of Occupational Safety and Health, some 900 were identified as toxic.

Note: 95% are derived from petroleum-based petrochemicals synthesized after World War II.

A report released by Coming Clean, the Environmental Working Group and Health Care Without Harm details a toxic family of chemicals known as **phthalates** (THAY-lates) which are found in everything from car parts to cosmetics especially beauty products like nail polish, lipstick, moisturizers and perfumes. The European Commission has recently proposed a ban on the uses of **phthalates** found in some of the world's best-known perfumes and cosmetics (Tommy Girl Perfume, Sure Ultra Deodorant, Vidal Sassoon) for causing infertility in men and genital abnormalities.

Phthalates are solvents used to help prevent the loss of fragrance in the products. They are endocrine **disruptors and block male hormones and feminize boys or contribute to male reproductive problems.** Cases of testicular cancer in young men have risen tenfold in the past century. Numerous animal studies have shown that phthalate exposures cause genital abnormalities (Sunday Times, Lois Rogers, November 25, 2002).

- From a sample of 1,029 people, every person tested showed positive for **phthalates** in their blood or urine.
- Scientists at the Centers for Disease Control singled out a particularly high incidence of **phthalates** amongst women of childbearing age.
- These women were found to have daily exposures of **phthalates** ranging from **2.5 to 22 times the normal for the rest of the general population,** with 5 percent showing levels of 75 percent or higher of the acceptable daily amounts.

- A study of New York City students presented online by Scientific American on January, 2010 found that **phthalate exposure** was linked to behavioral problems. The study pointed out that Children exposed in the womb to chemicals in cosmetics and fragrances are more likely to develop behavioral problems commonly found in children with attention deficit disorders.

- The research involved 188 children between the ages of 4 and 9 who were born between 1998 and 2002, according to the study published online in the journal **Environmental Health Perspectives**. Most were from East Harlem or the Upper East Side of Manhattan, and three-quarters of them were low-income.

- Nearly every human tested has traces of phthalates in his or her body and women are most highly exposed. *"There is sufficient evidence to be concerned about phthalates and it's prudent to reduce exposure as much as possible,"* Engel a Mount Sinai associate professor of preventive medicine and lead author of the study, said. *"But they are so ubiquitous right now it's hard to eliminate exposure without regulatory action."*

- The study points out that in a study published in 2009, Korean researchers linked childhood exposure to phthalates to ADHD.

- Engel said people should "press legislators" to restrict **phthalates** in adult, as well as children's, personal care products. The study has uncovered a new problem in impacting child neurodevelopment. Fetuses are *"uniquely vulnerable, particularly for endocrine disruptors,"* she said. *"But we are very concerned about the problem of post-natal exposure as well. The kids continue to be exposed as they grow up."* This is certainly true as phthalates are often used in cosmetics because they help retain fragrances and help lotions penetrate the skin.

Obviously, the continued uses of phthalates as with the other toxic chemicals are a quicker way to one's grave—hence I like to call these chemicals the **'grave diggers.'**

Some of the other toxic chemicals used in products especially in fragrancing, include: **toluene, ethanol, acetone, formaldehyde, limonene, benzene derivatives, methylene chloride, musk amberette, musk xylene, musk ketone, phenoxyethanol** and many others known to cause cancer, birth defects, infertility, kidney damage, nervous system damage and other symptoms.

For example, synthetic musk fragrance (about 8,000 tons are produced annually) is shown to have a carcinogenic effect in laboratory mice and to cause genetic damage in animal experiments plus other symptoms. They are ecologically harmful due to their high dermal permeability in animals and aquatic wildlife.

Every time you reach for the bottle of fragrant shampoo, soap or cologne, you are contaminating yourself and the environment- *how sanitary is it to wash with engine degreaser or antifreeze* under your armpits and on your teeth?

Would you eat butylated hydroxyl toluene (BHT) or stearmidopropyl dimethylamine for breakfast? Or rubbing formaldehyde into your hair and onto your skin?

Your skin eats too!

So every topical application of any soap, cosmetic, make-up etc. loaded with these chemicals is being fed to your skin. Redefining aging is also learning to choose wellness, which means knowing how to avoid the assaults and navigate wisely through the myriad of toxic chemicals.

FORMALDEHYDE: A MOST DANGEROUS SUBSTANCE

Formaldehyde is a colorless, flammable, strong-smelling gas chemical that is used in building materials and to produce many household and personal care products. It presents a health hazard if workers are exposed to it or if homeowners are exposed to it when new homes or building materials such as particleboard, plywood, and fiberboard; glues and adhesives; permanent-press fabrics; paper product coatings; are off-gassing. You can be exposed to formaldehyde if you breathe it into your lungs, if it gets into your eyes, or if it is contained in a product that gets onto your skin, like a perfume or a hair care product.

Formaldehyde is known to cause cancer. Dr. Samuel Epstein describes Formaldehyde as *"probably the most dangerous substance on the market."* It has been given a red flag by health agencies, yet this toxicant is still being used in **toiletries, cosmetics and dishwashing products.**

You can also be exposed to it accidentally if you touch your face, eat food, or drink after using a product containing formaldehyde without first washing your hands. The Occupational Safety & Health Administration site (OSHA) point out that formaldehyde can irritate the eyes and nose and cause coughing and wheezing. It is known as a "sensitizer," which means that it can cause allergic reactions of the skin, eyes, and lungs such as asthma-like breathing problems and skin rashes and itching. When formaldehyde is in a product that gets sprayed into the eyes, it can damage the eyes and cause blindness.

The (OSHA) website lists the dangers of formaldehyde along with the various other names or words for formaldehyde that are listed on the label instead. Unfortunately, many of these alternate names will not be recognized by the majority of the population.

Formaldehyde can be listed as **methylene glycol**, **formalin**, **methylene oxide**, **paraform**, **formic aldehyde**, **methanal**, **oxomethane**, **oxymethylene**, or **CAS Number 50-00-0**. All of these are names for formaldehyde under OSHA's Formaldehyde standard. There are other chemicals, such as timonacic acid (also called thiazolidinecarboxylic acid) that can release formaldehyde under certain conditions, such as those present during the hair smoothing treatment process.

"FRAGRANCE", "PERFUME" OR "PARFUM"

According to the Journal of the American College of Toxicology, "fragrance" could be any combination of more than **3,000 different synthetic chemical ingredients**. Chemical fragrances pose a serious health risk and are a significant source of indoor air pollution.

> According to the Journal of the American College of Toxicology, "fragrance" could be any combination of more than 3,000 different synthetic chemical ingredients.

This next section was taken from my ***Vibrational Cleaning*** book as it is worthwhile to present here: *A wide range of mainstream fragrances and perfumes, predominantly based on synthetic ingredients, are used in numerous cosmetics, toiletries, soaps and other household products. They are loaded with toxic and often carcinogenic compounds, including **formaldehyde**, toluene, phthalates and synthetic musk. Because manufacturers are allowed to guard their special blend of fragrance as a trade secret, none of these 3,000+ chemicals EVER get listed on the label.*

*"Currently, **the fragrance industry is virtually unregulated. Its recklessness is abetted and compounded by FDA's complicity.** The FDA has refused to require the industry to disclose ingredients due to trade secrecy considerations."*

No wonder so many people have developed allergies to smells (including myself)—as they are all fakes, mimickers and toxic ingredients. These chemicals that target the brain and the nervous system are called neurotoxins and they have created the 'environmental sensitivities' that have become more pervasive amongst the population. As a result, a real smell—e. g., a plant or a flower smell, or a non-adulterated essential oil—is now interpreted by the brain as an attack! These neurotoxic chemicals have distorted our endocrine, hormonal systems as well as our brain chemistry and memory. The system does not distinguish a safe smell to a toxic poisonous chemical. So the brain and nervous system reacts to all smells. To correct this sad state of affairs takes time, understanding, direction and dedication toward healthy living and aging which this guide is meant to assist with.

Debra Lynn Dadd an internationally-recognized consumer advocate specializing in identifying toxic products had this to say about neurotoxins:

"Neurotoxins are so called because they are toxic to your nervous system. The core of your nervous system is your brain, which not only affects thinking and feeling but regulates every system in your body. When your nervous system is damaged, your entire body can be affected."

OTHER MORE COMMON HARMFUL INGREDIENTS TO AVOID IN PARTICULAR ARE:

Alcohol – may increase risk of oral tongue and throat cancer. More men are diagnosed with oral and pharyngeal cancers (30,800 new cases diagnosed in 2002). Most commonly used in **mouthwashes.**

Aluminum – is a skin irritant and is linked to nerve damage, brain disorders, namely Alzheimer's. Mostly found in **deodorants.**

DEA (diethanolamine)/TEA – foam boosting surfactant emulsifier and dyeing aid. A potential carcinogen as previously discussed. Mostly found in **shampoos, conditioners, bubble bath, shaving gels, shower gels and cosmetics.**

Propylene Glycol (antifreeze solvent) – has been shown to cause dermatitis, kidney and liver abnormalities in animal studies and to inhibit skin cell growth. Warnings are listed on industrial bottles to avoid skin contact. Found in **deodorants, cosmetics, shaving gels, conditioners, shampoos, toothpaste, face creams.** (See chart for more detailed toxic effects.)

Read your Labels!

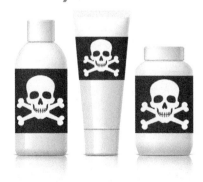

Sodium Lauryl Sulphate (engine degreaser) – may cause inflammation to the skin. SLS may damage children's teeth, mimics estrogens thus causing endocrine disruption, causes hair loss, and builds up in the heart, liver, lungs and brain. SLS can retard healing, cause cataracts and mouth ulcers. Found in **shampoos, toothpaste, mouthwash, hand creams, cleansers.** (See chart for more detailed toxic effects.)

Talc – linked to ovarian cancer. It is similar chemically to asbestos, a known cancer causing substance found in **body and baby powders, feminine powders and many cosmetics.** Commercial talcum powders contain an average of 19% of the asbestos-like mineral fibers namely, tremolite, anthophyllite and chrysotile. These fibers and particles are microscopic, and can permanently and easily lodge into the lungs reducing one's breathing. These particles can lead to asthmatic episodes. Women who used talc powder in the genital area had an increased ovarian cancer risk of 60% and women who used feminine deodorant sprays had a 90% increased risk (study in the **American Journal of Epidemiology**). These small particles seem to migrate into the female ovaries. Ovarian cancer is the fourth deadliest women's cancer in the U.S. Approximately 23,000 women were affected, killing 14,000 in 2001. Recent studies in the U.S. have conclusively found that frequent talcum powder usage in the genital area increases a woman's risk of developing ovarian cancer (Epstein 2001:160).

Diazo-lidinyl urea – a pesticide derived from alcohol. Used as a cosmetic preservative. It may release toxic formaldehyde, extremely common in personal care products. It falls under the category of "**formaldehyde doner" preservatives.**

Methyl-paraben – a preservative and germ fighter. Often causes allergic reactions.

Propyl-paraben – a popular, heavily used preservative to kill bacteria and fungi in the cosmetic industry. It's used in an estimated 13,200 cosmetic and skin care products. Studies implicate their connection with cancer due to the estrogen–mimicking quality and are thus disruptive to your endocrine system. Traces of parabens have been found in breast tumor samples. Parabens also often cause skin problems.

A study published in the Archives of Environmental Health found that certain fragrance fumes produced combinations of sensory irritation, pulmonary irritation, neuro toxic effects and allergic reactions. So it's not a surprise that asthma has increased in the last decade by 58% and that 72% of asthmatics have adverse reactions to fragrances. Once fragrances become airborne, they are easily inhaled by everyone in the surrounding area—it's the chemicals that linger on and cause the irritations. Many of the chemicals used to make gasoline and cigarettes are used to manufacture fragrances.

One survey of 14,000 pregnant women at the University of Bristol found that women exposed to aerosol deodorizers and air fresheners experienced headaches and depression, and the babies suffered from ear infections and diarrhea. Unfortunately, **there is no regulation in the fragrance industry,** even though chemicals in perfume are as damaging to health as tobacco smoke (WDDTY, Vol. 10 #7/99)!

Fragrances, when inhaled, no matter what their source, enter the blood stream and are able to breach the blood-brain barrier gaining access to the limbic system. This affects the emotional switchboard altering moods, affecting behavior and triggering depression.

In a 1991 report by America's environmental protection Agency (EPA), toluene was found (common chemical used in preparation of perfumes) in every single fragrance sample collected by the agency.

Toluene – is designated as a hazardous waste by the EPA and is a volatile petrochemical solvent and paint thinner. It has been shown to cause cancer and nervous system damage. It is also an endocrine disruptor. It is highly used in **fragrances, as well as in cosmetics and nail polish.** Toluene is a potent neurotoxicant that acts as an irritant, impairs breathing and causes nausea. Mothers' exposure to toluene vapors during pregnancy may cause developmental damage in the fetus. In human epidemiological studies and in animal studies toluene has also been associated with toxicity to the immune system and a possible link to blood cancer such as malignant lymphoma (EWG).

It is not surprising why the number of people reacting to perfumes has escalated with this potent neurotoxicant solvent. Reactions such as headaches, watery eyes, moodiness, tiredness, depression, irritability are a few of the reported symptoms. I do not find anything romantic about dabbing on hazardous waste onto your skin or exposing yourself to tobacco smoke and toxic vapors that cause cancer in mice! **Ninety percent of the EPA's hazardous waste list** was discovered in 10 well-known scented products – e.g. Chantilly spray mist, Giorgio perfume and Downy fabric softener. How does this all impact us? The body is estimated to absorb up to 5 Lbs of Make-Up Chemicals Per Year!

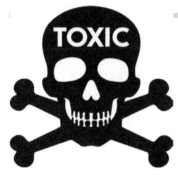

When you put these chemicals on your skin, it is worse than ingesting the toxins—why?

- These toxic chemicals are absorbed straight into your blood stream without filtering of any kind, so there's no protection against the toxins going directly to your delicate organs!

More is listed below on the two most common ingredients: Sodium Lauryl Sulphate and Propylene Glycol that are used in hundreds of personal care items. Remember: **Only 11% of 10,500 chemicals used in your cosmetics have been tested for safety!**

Whenever you buy a cosmetic or personal care product
READ THE LABEL!

See Appendix F Young Living Song

SODIUM LAURYL SULPHATE (SLS) USED AS:	PROPYLENE GLYCOL USED IN:

- Garage floor cleaner
- Engine degreaser
- Car wash detergents
- Shampoos with SLS could retard healing and keep children's eyes from developing properly in studies conducted at the University of Georgia (Green, et al., 1989). SLS is rapidly absorbed and accumulates in eye tissue being retained for up to 5 days. Children under six are especially vulnerable to improper eye development.
- Can cause cataracts in adults and delays healing of wounds in the surface of the cornea.
- Can cause skin to flake, separate and cause substantial roughness on the skin; used in clinical studies to irritate skin tissue.
- Is so caustic, it corrodes the hair follicle and impairs its ability to grow hair.

- Antifreeze
- Brake and hydraulic fluid
- Airplane de-icer
- Paint and coatings
- Floor wax
- Portable water systems
- Swimming pools
- Liquid laundry detergents
- Pet food and tobacco
- Propylene glycol serves as a humectant—a substance that helps retain moisture and hence its use in cosmetics, beauty creams, make-up & personal care items
- It is also found in children's personal care products.
- A clinical review in January 1991 American Academy of Dermatologists Inc. reported propylene glycol to cause a significant number of reactions and is a primary irritant to the skin even in low levels of concentration.
- Damages cell membranes causing rashes, dry skin and surface damage to the skin.
- May be harmful by inhalation, ingestion or skin absorption.
- May cause eye and skin irritation.
- Can cause gastro-intestinal disturbances, nausea, headache, and vomiting and central nervous system depression.

OUR SKIN— A HOLISTIC APPROACH

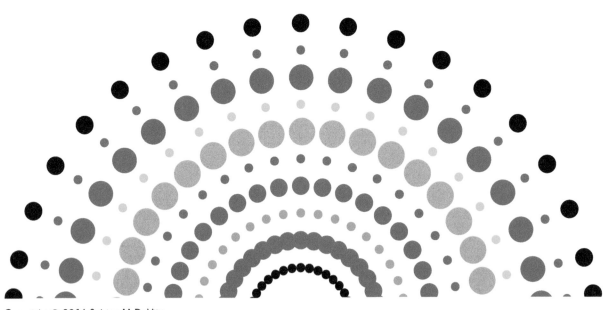

"Skin is alive and lifeless
chemicals cannot give life back to the skin."
PRATIMA RAICHUR/COHN, 1997

Our skin is as vital as our heart and lungs and is very much alive. Our skin breathes too; the skin directly absorbs up to 2.5% of the body's total oxygen requirement from the environment and expels 3% of the body's carbon dioxide waste. (Bharadwaj, 2000) What we put on our skin influences this vital exchange to breathe and if hampered in any way by chemical contaminants, the skin's function, condition and appearance are greatly compromised. The skin is also highly permeable to carcinogenic and toxic ingredients. **Women in particular** are at higher risk for absorption than men, as they are **more thin-skinned with more fat under their skin which accumulates bio-hazardous chemicals.** This makes women's skin more permeable, thus more susceptible to transdermal passage of toxic chemicals and other foreign substances.

There is evidence showing that the permeability of skin to carcinogens may be greater than that of the intestines. As presented at the 1978 congressional hearings, the absorption of nitrosodiethanolamine (NDELA) formed by nitrosation of DEA is over **100 times greater** from the skin than by mouth. Consumption of this carcinogen has been associated with up to four- and seven-fold increased risks of childhood brain cancer and leukemia (S. Epstein)!

Some 30 U.S. and international studies have confirmed the high incidence of concerns in children whose parents were exposed to a variety of chemical carcinogens in the workplace during pregnancy. The FDA warned that a high percentage of cosmetics and personal care products contain carcinogenic nitrosamine contaminants.

Over 30 years ago, Rachel Carson's book called **Silent Spring** first warned us of the deadly toll that synthetic chemicals were taking on birds and wildlife. Today, the ground breaking work by Theo Colborn et. al., in **Our Stolen Future** gives us an utterly gripping account that traces birth defects, sexual abnormalities and reproductive failures in wildlife to the countless man-made chemical compounds never encountered before. These chemicals containing similar shapes to hormone molecules disrupt the functions normally controlled by the endocrine system and are now labeled as endocrine disrupter chemicals or **"gender benders."** We face a serious situation today. There is a wide spread use of dangerous compounds in our total environment: over **100,000 synthetic chemicals** are now on the market around the world that includes a wide range of industrial carcinogens (persistent organic pollutants or POPs) like organochlorine pesticides. Since 1965, more than **4 million** distinct chemical compounds have been formulated. At least **250,000 new formulations** are created annually. Over **800 neurotoxic chemical** compounds have been used in the cosmetic and perfume industries.

According to an EWG (Environmental Working Group) 2004 consumer survey, it showed that while on average women use 12 personal care products daily, men use an average of six a day, women expose themselves to more than **80 unique ingredients**. So, it's important to know your products and your ingredients!

The chemical pollutants have increased over the years, mainly because we were duped into believing they were safe, only to discover that they have been making us ill, aging us and causing premature death. The EPA issued a warning that simple contact with petrochemical toxins is enough to get them into your bloodstream. *"In just 26 seconds after exposure to chemicals, they can be found in every organ in the body"* (Published flyer "Top 10 'Killer' Household Chemicals"). **60 percent of whatever is applied to the skin gets absorbed into it!**

We can do something about this "chemical soup" by knowing that our pocket book holds the power. We have the ultimate choice in our choice of products and what we buy. We must do everything in our charge to return to a more natural way of living and one that is more sensible or a **'scents-able' way of life**. In so doing, we will have a better chance to live longer, younger and healthier. The simple answer in being "scents-able" embraces our ancestry in natural, holistic living. Natures' own plant factory of essential oils has a much safer track record that Chapter 6 will outline further.

THE ANTI-AGING BOOM: WHAT IS THE COST?

The increasing trend in longevity and anti-aging procedures continues to rise more than ever. As pointed out earlier, our society is consumed with youthfulness and beauty. Dozens of new formulas to stop aging are placed on the market weekly! As Pratima Raichur, co-author with M. Cohn, and a naturapathic/ayurvedic physician, states in their book, **Absolute Beauty,** *"For decades, Americans have spent billions of dollars annually, looking for the next 'magic' skin care ingredient, and we still have not found one"* (1997, page 6).

There are more statistics to add to those already presented in the introductory chapter. According to the American Society for Aesthetic Plastic Surgery (ASAPS), a **228 percent**

increase in the overall cosmetic (surgical and non-surgical) procedures has occurred since 1997. In 2000, approximately 7.4 million Americans had cosmetic surgery, mostly done **by women who spend $20 billion a year to improve wrinkles.** Canadian figures by the Canadian Society of Plastic Surgeons approximate about 740,000. More than one million men underwent cosmetic enhancement.

The most common non-surgical and seemingly popular procedure in 2002 was botulinum toxin injection (BOTOX). Botox injections have increased some 2,400 percent since 1997 way beyond what Dr. Oz presented. It seems quite ironic that a most powerful poison known to humanity is being used for so-called '"Beauty" (See "Beauty by Lethal Injection"—highlighted later in this chapter). Botulism is among the most severe types of food poisoning one can obtain, affecting the central nervous system. The toxins block the the transmission of nerves to muscles, thus paralyzing the muscles.

Early symptoms of botulism include extreme weakness, arrhythmia, double vision, coronary artery disturbances, thyroid dysfunction, droopy eyelids and trouble swallowing, leading to paralysis and death in severe cases. (ASAPS) reports that although Botox is generally safe, botulinum toxin **side effects and complications** can include:

- Bruising and pain at the injection site
- Flu-like symptoms
- Headache
- Nausea
- Redness
- Temporary facial weakness or drooping
- Very rarely, the toxin can spread beyond the treatment area, which can cause botulism like signs and symptoms such as breathing problems, trouble swallowing, muscle weakness, and slurred speech.

Botox is so deadly that germ warfare experts fear it as a weapon of terror. It works by paralyzing the muscles, making the wrinkles disappear temporarily. It lasts for only a few months (at a price on average of $400 per treatment) only to be repeated several times a year and several thousands of dollars later. Botulinum toxin can be used to help smooth:

- Crow's feet
- Forehead furrows
- Frown lines
- Skin bands on the neck

Other new uses introduced for Botulinum toxin include **reduction in sweating of hands and armpits (hyperhydrosis) and relief of headaches.** The latest rave in Botox use has recently been made available as a facial firming serum called A-Tox. The serum was developed for those individuals who dislike needles and introduced into the market in 2003 (Time, February 2003)! The serum is readily available today by various outlets. Cosmetic companies are hawking similar products, sold worldwide, called "Wrinkletox" and "Biotoc."

What has our world come to in the name of Beauty! Wouldn't this poison seep into the rest of the body over time, leading to later illness? The war on wrinkles continues to expand with other popular procedures: Often referred to as "The Quick Fixes" for the face:

a) Fillers – the most common is collagen (sterilized bovine collagen) injected under the skin to plump up or reduce the wrinkles. The benefits are temporary: the collagen is absorbed by the skin in anywhere from three months to two years. Some doctors are concerned that the repeated injections might compromise the body's immune defense system and lead to later illness.

Beauty By Lethal Injection!

Dermatologists have hatched up the perfect treatment—they inject a person with the deadly poison that causes the often-fatal food poisoning disease —botulism. The poison paralyzes the facial nerves, thus removing or softening the lines on wrinkled faces. And if the dermatologist were ever to become over excited and inject below the nose, the mouth could be permanently paralyzed but this area would be free of wrinkles!

(WDDTY, Vol. 10, No. 1/99)

b) Laser resurfacing – the skin is vaporized with a beam of intense light and heat. This moderately burns the skin so that it heals like new. It leaves skin raw and red for weeks.

c) Microdermabrasion – is a procedure where the skin is resurfaced (more like sanded) by a stream of aluminum oxide or salt with a rotating abrasive tool that removes the top layer of skin, revealing smoother, fresher skin underneath. It can also be used to rid scars and tattoos.

d) Chemical peels – mild to strong solutions are used (usually acids like lactic, glycolic and salicylic) to chemically peel the skin's outer layer. This is often drastic and harsh on sensitive skin. Furthermore, alpha-hydroxy acid has devastating health effects known to most consumers. They make the user more sensitive to ultraviolet radiation from sunlight which can cause skin cancer (Dr. Epstein).

Botox Deficiency? Sounds absurd . . . but that is what the beauty industry promotes with its Botox injections or creams. Instead you need to ask the most important question about what is the cause of frown lines, wrinkles, bags under the eyes, sagging skin and any of the other 'aging signs' in the first place.

MORE BEAUTY FILLERS!

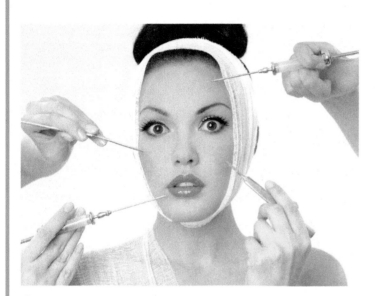

Now there are more fillers on the market!

Time's article (May 19, 2003) **Beyond Botox** reports how recently developed *"injectable wrinkle busters"* are flooding *the New market for wrinkles.*

Botox is wonderful for the forehead and crow's feet but not for the lower face so this has fueled the desire for other fillers. Here are the witches' brews of injectables:

Cow collagen, liquid silicone, plastic micro beads, synthetic bone, synthetic hyaluronic acid and ground-up skin of human cadavers! Wow! how outrageous is that but as shocking as it is, some people will do whatever it takes for beauty!

Unfortunately, our culture has jumped onto the bandwagon for a "quick fix" which focuses only on treating symptoms that are often dangerous, temporary, toxic and expensive. It has also lost sight of the true meaning of the word **"cosmetics."**

THE HOLISTIC APPROACH: WE'RE CONNECTED

"The body and mind are one.
When the intimate relationship between mind
and body is disrupted, aging and entropy accelerate."
DEEPAK CHOPRA

TRUE MEANING OF COSMETICS: WHAT IS BEAUTY?

For the Greeks, the creation of the world (or universe) was the creation of order (the kosmos) out of chaos (Kaos). Thus the universe is "the Order": or the Cosmos which is fundamentally beautiful. The more ordered the cosmos, the closer it is to the 'Dea' who is the Divine Beauty.

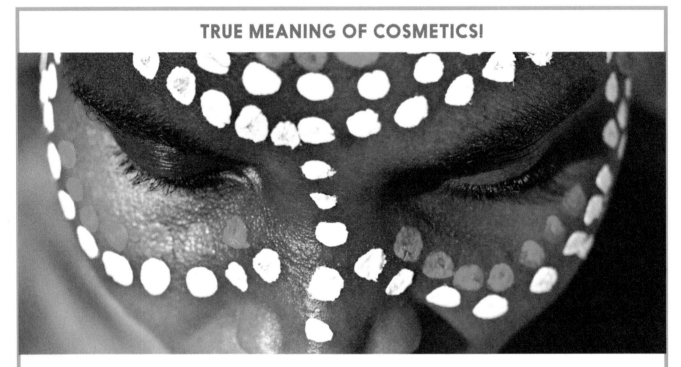

TRUE MEANING OF COSMETICS!

*Cosmetics are one of the most ancient arts known to humanity. It is interesting to note that "**cosmetics**" comes from the Greek word "**kosmetikos**" which actually means "**skill in arranging.**" The root word "kosmos" means 'order.' In its traditional sense beauty meant,* "Harmonizing your lifestyle as well as bringing order to the mind and inner workings of the body" (Sachs, 1994, page 155).

Thus it was viewed that all earthly beauty is a fragment or reflection of the Divine Beauty. The absolute Beauty is the source and wellspring of the beauty in every beautiful thing we see about us.

When we seek to enhance and make the most of feminine beauty on earth, what we are in fact doing is pursuing an ancient art which is literally, spiritual, in bringing more 'order', or bringing ourselves into alignment with the Cosmos itself, by maximising our small part in its order and beauty. Today's understanding of this root definition has been unfortunately lost.

What happened to this inner wisdom and knowledge? Beautiful, radiant and youthful skin can only be obtained by adhering to a healthy, orderly, holistic and natural lifestyle. There is no quick fix. As author, filmmaker Markus Rothkranz states in his book: `Heal Your Face` `The answer is not painting over rust, but finding out what caused the rust in the first place.``(2011, p.9)

Also, Beauty can be seen as a perfection of order or rhythm.

Walter Russell, artist, architect, author & philosopher, states beauty as "Perfection of rhythm, balanced perfection of rhythm. Everything in Nature is expressed by rhythmic waves of light. Every thought and action is a light-wave of thought and action."

The mind and body are inseparable, they are one. As Deepak Chopra (2001) states in his book, **Grow Younger, Live Longer,** that "Wherever a thought goes, a chemical goes with it." We're connected. A new Western science called **psychoneuroimmunology** that has developed over the last twenty years endorses this philosophy that the mind and body are one. It simply states that our mind and emotions (the way we think and how we feel) profoundly influence our physical well being. They are not inseparable. The term Psychoneuroimmunology was coined in 1975 by Dr. Robert Ader, director of the division of behavioral and psychosocial medicine at New York's University of Rochester. Dr. Ader believed that there is a link between what we think (our state of mind) and our health and our ability to heal ourselves.

The resarch in Psychoneuroimmunology has shown that **various attitudes and emotional reactions in the human body directly affect the immune system.** Dr. Chopra refers to the immune system listening in to our thoughts. For example, the endocrine system weakens when there is a dominance of repressed, bottled up toxic emotions such as pain, anger and fear. However, it is stimulated or enhanced when there is an increase of such positive emotions as pleasure and love. **Evidence shows that our emotions and thoughts "talk" with the billions of defense cells in our immune system.** Happy thoughts create a happy, healthy, well-functioning immune system.

It has taken medicine three hundred years to finally awaken this truth of "whole-ism" (holistic). We can give thanks to the scientific genius of Albert Einstein, who believed in "nature's inherent harmony." He changed science and medicine forever when he initiated the theory of relativity and quantum theory. Albert Einstein's famous equation E=MC2 has given us the key insight toward understanding that **energy and matter are**

interchangeable. In other words, all matter is in constant motion and that matter itself is, in fact, vibrating energy (known as "chi" or prana) energy that vibrates at different frequencies. Dr. Richard Gerber in **Vibrational Medicine** refers to humans as multi-dimensional "beings of energy" and that *"energy and matter are dual expressions of the same universal substance."* We are one, indivisible dynamic whole whose parts are interrelated.

This concept is not new. The Greek physician, Galen, in 200 A.D. commented on how cancer seemed to afflict melancholic women more frequently than those that were happy (Epstein, 1998). Scientists today are acknowledging that our immune system is profoundly affected by our emotions. According to Dr. Candace Pert, a neuroscientist, neuro-pharmacologist, biochemist, author of **Molecules of Emotion**, points out those **bodily emotions are the key**, *"Emotions are the nexus between mind and matter, going back and forth between the two and influencing both."* Her audio entitled, **Your Body Is Your Subconscious Mind**, summarizes her discoveries as she says, *"Consciousness creates reality—that is the central principle."*

The natural chemical messengers, called Neuropeptides, were at one time thought to be found in the brain alone. Pioneering research by Candace Pert revealed that these neuropeptides are present on both the cell walls of the brain and in the immune system. These information substances affect our emotions as well as our physiology.

Dr. Bruce Lipton author of **Biology of Belief** an internationally recognized, quantum biologist and authority in bridging science and spirit revealed a 'new biology' that has revolutionized scientific thinking when he pointed out that it's our mind that controls our genetic expression.

In other words, our cells and our DNA are more influenced by our thoughts, our beliefs and our imagination than anything else around us. Our minds have the power to create or cure disease and create beautiful skin because our thoughts affect the expression of our genes. This new field in genetics, as discovered by Dr. Bruce Lipton, is called "Epi-genetics" which shows how our environment dictates and shapes our DNA. He points out that our state of health is dictated far more by our beliefs and our attitudes than by our genes. The role of these environmental toxins (be it food toxins, heavy metals, cosmetic toxins, stress, our words, etc.) is what shapes our DNA. So simply put looking younger is a **holistic concept**. The next chapter expands on the role of Stress and research discoveries.

This body-mind notion was well-known by the ancient wisdom of the world's oldest system of health care and healing, called Ayurveda. Ayurveda, derived from two sanskrit roots, **Ayus, meaning "life"** and **Veda, meaning "science"** or **"Immortality,"** is often referred to as India's traditional medicine.

Ayurveda promotes longevity without limit based on the belief that life is immortal: it embraces a wholesome lifestyle, diet and a positive mental attitude. It is also based on the premise that the mind and the body are unified on the level of consciousness – and for six thousand years has emphasized the causative role of thought and behavior in health and disease. Thus, the Ayurvedic practitioner identifies skin problems as a symptom of a disturbance of the whole person. This philosophy is totally unlike what Western medicine still adheres to, by treating skin symptoms in isolation using toxic and invasive approaches as I outlined in the previous section on the "Anti-Aging Boom." Dr. Chopra reminds us that, *"viewing your body from the perspective of quantum physics opens up new modes of understanding and experiencing the body and its aging. The practical essence of this new understanding is that human beings can reverse their aging"* (2001, Page 12).

Ayurveda delineates all phenomena into a simple framework for understanding life, creation, mind and matter. Similar to the traditional Chinese system, all existence is an interplay of two cosmic forces in which yin and yang are eternally changing, transforming and balancing. Old Chinese philosophers conceived the whole universe to be filled with a vital energy called "chi," known as "prana" in the Ayurvedic system.

Everything that exists is classified into five categories (the "chi" energy or "prana" being manifested into the physical) known as the Five Elements—Fire, Earth, Metal (Air – Ayurvedic), Water, Wood (Space – Ayurvedic).

These five elements in nature are the first objective expressions of consciousness. They give rise to the five senses: they combine to create all the forms and functions of one's psychophysiology—in other words, one's nature or constitution. According to Ayurveda, all experiences are understood in terms of the interaction of the elements. The elements in combination give rise to three biological forces or principles called "Tridoshas"—three humors or temperaments known as:

Vata – made up of both air and ether (space) elements

Pitta – fire and water elements

Kapha – earth and water elements

The three doshas, or constitutions, are the dynamic movements of life—inertia, excitability and equilibrium—defined as "unbound intelligence" (Raichur/Cohn, 1997). According to Ayurveda, each individual has a unique proportion of the three constitutions, or doshas, and can be classified as Vata (air and ether), Pitta (fire and water) and Kapha (earth and water) type or temperament.

These five elements, similar to Chinese system of diagnosis, are always present within us mentally, physically and emotionally. The "doshas" or elements become imbalanced at times due to stress, seasonal changes, diet, emotional trauma, poor lifestyle habits or chemical/environmental toxins, leading to disorder (out of order or chaos) or disease. When the system is imbalanced, the skin is affected.

In the Ayurvedic system, the goal is to restore balance to the elements and then to the skin—this restores the flow of intelligence to the body, mind and spirit. The elements must be maintained in order to stay youthful and healthy.

In **Absolute Beauty**, Dr. Pratima Raichur states, for example, that in order to treat acne, we need to first eliminate the physical and emotional imbalances that weakened the body's immunity which enabled the bacteria to negatively affect the skin, causing acne. This holistic approach has been Ayurveda's message for six thousand years. It supports the body's natural, inherent wisdom and abilities to balance itself—by the right diet, breathing, thinking, emotional flow, exercise, proper nutritionals and the life-giving ingredients for the skin that are only found from Mother Nature's own pharmacopoeia, the plants, pure extracts or essential oils. Similarly, Markus Rothkranz in **Heal Your Face** also points out that every part of your face is connected to a different and specific part of your body. Your face reflects the condition of your internal organs. For example, lines running from your nose to the sides of your mouth are an indicator of a clogged colon and/or general weakness (See Appendix E).

Today we have the means to measure the various emotional, mental and physical imbalances. Dr. Konstantin Korotkov, Professor of Physics at St. Petersburg State Technical University in Russia, scientist, author, researcher on the Human Energy Field, developed the Gas Discharge Visualization Kirlian camera (GDV), as a way to measure the energy field. It is a breakthrough technology beyond Kirlian photography for direct, real-time viewing of the human field or aura. This new technology allows one to capture by a special camera the physical, emotional, mental and spiritual energy emanating to and from an individual; the energy field reflects the state of one's consciousness on different levels. The GDV Kirlian is the most accurate device in the world to visually show one's subconscious blueprint. In other words, the content of our energy field or Aura determines our reality (See chapter 14 for more information and GDV pictures).

With so much emphasis in our society on youth and beauty, many women today become clouded with the latest trends. Besides the thrust in chemical "fixes," another recent trend is in the use of **cosmeceuticals** that target the symptoms of aging skin. While cosmeceuticals are somewhat better in some of their ingredients than the chemical skin care products by utilizing some nutritive compounds, they still feature isolated active ingredients and can include toxic chemicals as well. One of the major concerns with cosmeceuticals today as stated by Dr. Epstein in chapter 1 is the use of **nano particles**. Research suggests that these tiny **nano particles** are highly dangerous, penetrate the skin and cause cell damage.

Essential oils are your best and safe way to nurture your skin. They embody the wholeness of the plant, working synergistically to support the overall health of the skin. The most expensive skin preparations on the world market today contain essential oils. Essential oils are powerful healing substances from nature containing the highest antioxidants naturally inherent in the constituents of the oils (more in Chapter 6). Essential oils support the overall health of the skin through a holistic approach by assisting the skin to perform its own natural functions. Essential oils are not a quick fix by any means, nor did anyone develop wrinkles overnight. It is a holistic lifestyle to radiant beauty and 'agelessness' aging.

"For every human illness, somewhere in the world
there exists a plant which is the cure."
RUDOLPH STEINER

'Beauty Is an inside job of an outside view.'
SABINA DEVITA

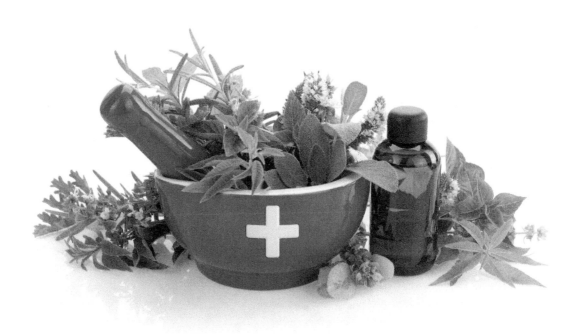

CHAPTER 4

CAUSES OF AGING SKIN

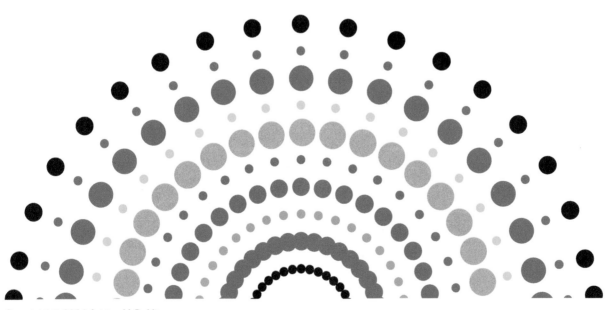

"When virtue and modesty enlighten her charms,
the lustre of a beautiful woman
is brighter than the stars of heaven
and the influence of her power
tis in vain to resist."
AKHENATON

ABOUT YOUR SKIN

The skin is the largest eliminative and most adaptable organ of the body. Its purpose is to protect against bacterial invasion and prevent dehydration. It is critical to detoxify the body through sweat and secretions. It also acts as a receptor for light that stimulates body functions. It is the body's first line of defense (the skin is the only organ that is constantly exposed to the environment—the elements) and can be easily damaged by external causes, sunlight and air pollution and internal ones.

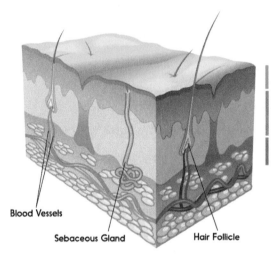

Epidermis

Dermis

Hypodermis

Blood Vessels

Sebaceous Gland

Hair Follicle

The skin readily shows the internal conditions of the organs as stated earlier and, in that sense; you cannot be in a healthy state on the inside if your skin looks rough, pasty, wrinkled and dehydrated on the outside. Literally, your face is a way of showing you what is going on inside you as each external part of your body and face is connected to an internal organ. This makes for an awesome immediate read-out of what is going on—without any expensive tests—it's your own diagnostic system.

Outside beauty is an inside job of maintaining healthy organs. The skin is also the major producer of endocrine hormones and vitamin D, which control most physiological functions. **A Fascinating Fact: It actually secretes more hormones than does the endocrine system itself** (Chopra, 2001, Raichur/Cohn 1997)! The skin is formed of three principal layers: epidermis, dermis, and fat layer or subdermis.

EPIDERMIS

This is the skin's outer layer comprised of keratinized, stratified epithelial tissue. The epidermis consists of two main cells—keratinocytes and melanocytes. The outer surface is called the stratum corneum, a protective coating of dead skin cells, thinner than a sheet of tissue paper, which helps the skin hold in moisture and oils. This outer layer is sloughed off continually when new skin cells form and push their way to the surface. **Epidermal cell productions normally regenerate every 27 days, and as we age, this slows down to twice the norm every 50 days.** Simply, we do not make new cells as quickly. The melanocytes, also part of the epidermis layer, produce melanin that determines the color of your skin. What it also means is that whatever was used and eaten 27–50 days ago will be evidenced or mirrored in your skin today.

DERMIS

This thick connective tissue makes up 90% of the thickness of your skin. It contains a dense network of collagen and elastin—two types of protein which gives the skin its strength, durability, resilience and elasticity. The dermis contains nerve receptors (your sensitivity to touch, pain, temperature) and sweat glands, sebaceous glands. The sweat and sebaceous glands help produce your skin's acid mantel as protection from infections. Harsh soaps often strip this away. During the ages of 40 to 50, the sweat glands decrease in size and number, the dermis loses cellular content, which impedes the blood flow, weakens the immune system, and the collagen fibers lose their strength and durability, causing the skin to sag (Raichur/Cohn 1997).

SUBDERMIS OR FAT CELLS

This is the deepest layer of the skin composed mainly of fat tissue, to insulate and protect your inner organs and helps keep the skin plump and smooth. All portions of the skin are provided with a system of lymphatic channels that supply the nutrients to the larger vessels beneath the skin. Lymph is abundantly supplied to the skin; some 60% of total—at least one liter and up to 2 gallons is evaporated off or perspired as sweat daily. Hence, the importance of drinking water. Dr. Bihova, co-author of **Beauty from the Inside Out** says, *"Healthy skin is about 10 to 20% water."* When skin loses more than half its moisture, it becomes dry and flaky and fine lines become more pronounced.

Dr. Whitaker also points out in 'Shed 10 Years In 10 Weeks' that skin ages because we lose water (skin loses about 30% of its water content). Thus skin becomes drier; we lose collagen—the mattress of the skin which begins to shrink; and we lose hormones which helps the skin to retain its moisture (more on hormones in Chapter 8).

"Aging is really about caring for worn-out parts."
SUZANNE SOMERS

THE YOUTH STEALERS AGE YOU FASTER

1. FREE RADICAL THEORY OR OXIDATIVE STRESS

A number of researchers including Dr. Whitaker present the free radical theory proposed by Den-ham Harman, Ph.D. back in the 1950s as the most widely accepted theory for aging. Simply stated, free radicals are oxygen molecules that have lost an electron in interactions with other molecules. In their quest to bind, they steal other electrons from healthy molecules creating more free radicals. As Dr. Perricone points out, collagen, a protein, gives our skin its youthful suppleness and tautness, and is especially susceptible to damage from free radicals. The free radical attack on the skin (most notably sun exposure) leads to a chemical change called cross-linking, which wreaks havoc on the protein molecules that make up our skin.

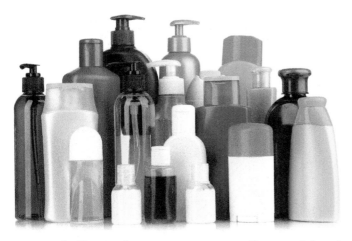

Our bodies are bombarded daily by free radicals. Dr. Bruce Ames, University of California, estimates that the DNA of each cell is attacked by free radicals over 10,000 times per day. One of the major ways we expose our skin to free radicals is in the use of synthetic cosmetics and toiletries. It is estimated that we rub (from the time we are babies to adulthood) **an estimated 2,000 liters (84,000 ounces) of chemical-based lotions, shampoos, cosmetics and body products into our skin more than 470,000 times** (Borkovic, 2003)!

Other researchers are discovering how devastating free radical damage can be to fats that form phospholipid membranes of almost every cell in the body. As cell membranes become less fluid, they lose their ability to function normally, hastening tissue and organ damage and lead to premature death. When there are more free radical atoms and/or molecules than antioxidants—(the regenerative and repair ability of the cells to neutralize them) we now have **Oxidative Stress!**

Cigarette smoking causes free radical production in the body and, at the same time, depletes antioxidants. A new study in 2014 reported that cigarette smoking causes accelerated Facial aging. **Smokers place themselves at a higher risk for oxidative stress.** Oxidative stress sets up the body for diseases like heart failure, cancer, Parkinson's etc.

In fact, studies show that FREE RADICALS in cells accelerates AGING, the problems associated with AGING and contributes to more than **200 HEALTH conditions.**

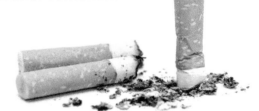

MANY STUDIES ARE ALSO REPORTING HOW TOXINS IN THE ENVIRONMENT MAY ACCELERATE AGING.

- Avoiding ***environmental toxins*** may be the key to preserving your youth, according to new research. So cleaning your home of these environmental contaminants may help to keep you younger as well!
- Experts now believe a class of environmental toxins—known as **gerontogens**—may put people at an increased risk for **accelerated aging.**

Toxins present in cigarette smoke, (published study Dec. 2013) UV rays and chemotherapy are all suspected **gerontogens**—capable of accelerating the rate at which a person ages. It's interesting to note that more women tend to stop smoking when they learn smoking greatly increases wrinkles (Pina LoGiudice ND, LAc and Peter Bongiorno ND, LAc Directors of Inner Source Health). The greatest "**anti**" or protection from free radicals are "**anti-oxidants.**" More on this is presented in Chapter 6.

2. METHYLATION

Another contributing factor to aging is called methylation. Dr. Whitaker describes this as cellular housekeeping, a crucial chemical reaction that occurs billions of times every second. That is the DNA within each cell requires certain enzymatic reactions to maintain youthful metabolism.

When methylation becomes inefficient and sluggish, toxic compounds build up like dust balls under the sofa. Most significant toxic compound is homocysteine, which can harm the arteries and impair circulation. It also damages the cell's DNA and contributes to arteriosclerosis, heart disease, stroke, Alzheimer's, cancer and other diseases of aging. Some of the housecleaning tools that are needed are vitamins B-6, B-12 and folic acid.

3. SUGAR AGES YOU – GLYCOSYLATION

This is a process caused by **sugar**, which binds and chemically alters the protein in the body. It occurs internally as well as in the skin. Sugar is exceptionally damaging to the skin because it attaches to the proteins of collagen, causing a break down or the collagen to cross-**link**. This makes the skin stiff and inflexible, causing wrinkling due to the buildup of advanced glycation end-products (AGEs). This cross-linkage occurs inside or outside the cell impairing the cell's functions that cause damage to it. Sadly, diabetics suffer accelerated glycation.

Keeping blood sugar levels in the normal range may retard Glycosylation. Steer clear of refined carbohydrates, sugar, sodas, cold cereals, and most bread and snack foods as they blast into the system and raise the blood sugar.

Blood sugar in the body can damage body tissues and contribute to aging. Blood sugar crystals are involved in glycation reactions: glycation reactions are basically reactions where the sugar melds with protein in our body tissues (like in blood vessels, for example) and breaks them down. This reaction creates Advanced Glycation End products (aptly called "AGEs") and is a major player in the aging of our tissues—and ages your body the way bread gets crusty. The more AGEs you have, the more you get "crusty" and age. These AGEs build up causing blood vessels to narrow, contributing to high blood pressure, vascular disease and heart attacks. AGEs are linked to insulin resistance, poor blood sugar control and the accumulation of damaging substances in the brain, including the plaques found in Alzheimer's brains. They have also been implicated in rheuma-toid arthritis, kidney disease and inflammatory bowel disorders (Suzanne Somers, **Bombshell**).

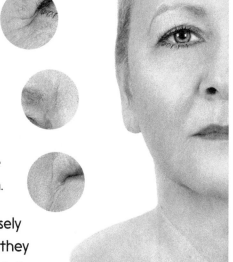

Of course, the way to limit the AGEs in our bodies is to limit or avoid any of the items mentioned previ-ously—that is any refined white sugar and any simple carbohydrates; avoid processed or any prepack-aged foods, fast foods and micro waved foods. Our society is built on the 'sweet tooth' phenomenon that so many prepared foods are loaded with sugars, such as ketchup or relish. Read your labels for any of these prepared foods, your salad dressings, sauces and so on.

Unfortunately, many more people have been falsely influenced to use **aspartame** instead, thinking that they are correcting one 'negative' with another. That is not the case—**aspartame is extremely toxic and dangerous** and is strongly linked to brain cancer and tumors. Once ingested, aspartame breaks down into formaldehyde (a well-known carcinogen presented earlier in this guidebook).

One nutrient well known to help with sugar cravings is GTF chromium. It helps to control the sugar spikes that can damage the inside vessels and the vessels that keep your skin looking young and vital. GTF chromium is naturally found in the food Brewer's yeast. An optimal dose of GTF chromium is 500 mcg (micrograms) once or twice a day.

Ajinomoto the company that makes Aspartame has given Aspartame a new-name due to its bad press as being dangerous. The name has been changed to AminoSweet but contains the same toxic ingredients.

What is most alarming as well is how it continues to gain approval for use in new types of food despite evidence showing that it causes neurological brain damage, cancerous tumors and endocrine disruption, among other harmful conditions. Aspartame is still being used as an everyday ingredient in most diet beverages, sugar-free desserts and chewing gums in countries worldwide.

James Schlatter, a chemist who had been trying to produce an anti-ulcer pharmaceutical drug for G.D. Searle & Company back in 1965 discovered Aspartame accidentally. Upon mixing aspartic acid and phenylalanine, two naturally-occurring amino acids, he discovered that the new compound had a sweet taste. The company merely changed its FDA approval application from drug to food additive and aspartame was born.

Aspartame is a carcinogen that was illegitimately approved as a food additive through heavy-handed prodding by a powerful corporation with its own interests in mind. What the general public is unaware of is that practically all drugs and food additives are approved by the FDA because companies essentially lobby the FDA with monetary payoffs and complete the agency's multi-million dollar approval process not because science shows they are safe! So don't be fooled when it comes to FDA approval.

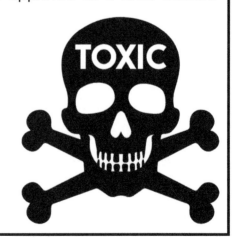

4. INFLAMMATION CONNECTION

Inflammation, known as swelling, is an integral part of the immune response. As we get older, the body's ability to remove by-products of inflammation is impaired. Inflammation takes place internally as well as externally. Particularly with the skin, it invites lines and wrinkles. Inflammatory chemicals called cytokines damage the cell and accelerates aging. Chronic inflammation is a more serious condition. It is involved in Alzheimer's and in type 2 diabetes.

essential oils have been found to preserve and protect the breakdown of EPA in the tissues.

Recent research has uncovered strong links between **chronic inflammation** and cardiovascular disease. Eliminating bad fats and increasing good ones helps to control inflammation. Eicosapentaenoic acid (EPA), a fatty acid found in fish oils, is very effective in controlling inflammation. Essential oils have also been found to act as anti-inflammatory agents quite successfully using similar mechanisms as EPA, and they are even more beneficial as essential oils have been found to preserve and protect the breakdown of EPA in the tissues. (Youdim and Deans, 1999)

Vitamin B6 is a major player in protecting the skin, as it converts Essential Fatty Acids (EFA) into active chemicals called prostaglandins. Prostaglandins do an excellent job of controlling the chemicals that cause inflammation. Vitamin B6 also helps to prevent heart disease. Since it is water-soluble, it needs to be replenished on a regular daily basis.

Wonderfully, Dr. Andrew Weil on *Healthy Aging: Your Online Guide to the Anti-Inflammatory Diet* provides in his online resource an Anti-Inflammatory Diet. He believes that the Anti-Inflammatory Diet can help people to age gracefully even delay the onset of age-related diseases and discomforts.

5. PSYCHO-PHYSIOLOGICAL ASPECTS

How Are You Handling Stress or Not?

There is another aspect dynamically involved in the aging of the skin which happens in the internal processes due to emotions, thoughts and **stress**. The psycho-physiological imbalances alter the function of individual skin cells and alter one's facial appearances. An old expression from the Ayurvedic system states, "To know a person's experiences from the past, examine their body now" (Chopra 2001). *Your face is an open book to the world. It is the mirror for what you are feeling and have been feeling.*

In *Why People Don't Heal and How They Can*, Carolyn Myss points out how our "**biography becomes our biology!**" Toxic emotions are like battery acid to the body and are often the most harmful accelerators in the aging process. Anger, resentment, fear, regret —all erode the life-force, upset one's equilibrium and disturbs the immune and hormonal systems. These imbalances cause one's sebaceous glands to produce excess oil, leading to rashes, spots and blotches. Have we not heard the expressions "it's written all over your face"? Or "what's got under your skin?" See chapter on energy psychology techniques to help to de-stress along with specific aromatic essential oils.

Stress is at an all time high globally. According to many physicians, stress has surpassed the cold virus as the most common health problem in North America. I believe this has led to the dangerous over prescribing of antidepressants in our society. Our generation is experiencing more stress today, than our forefathers ever did due to the massive increases of stressors in our everyday lives: immense busyness and demands in the work place, at home, financial-economic concerns, electromagnetic pollution exposures (cell phones, computers, power lines, cell towers, etc) alongside the everyday emotional stressors that people are contending with in their personal lives, plus the chemical onslaught as presented earlier. And to add to the list, humankind is overwhelmingly bombarded with world events: of strife, war, violence and other horrific calamities (nuclear radiation from Fukushima) and other on-going violent world threats.

The American Medical Association reports that nearly 80 percent of all diseases are either stress-related or stress antagonized. Dr. Bruce Lipton suggests that stress is associated with up to 90 percent of all conditions that send people to the doctor's office. Nearly 65 percent of adults report feeling under great stress and reports from the **American Institute of Stress** point out as many as 75 to 90 percent of all visits to primary-care physicians result from stress-related disorders (Childre and Martin).

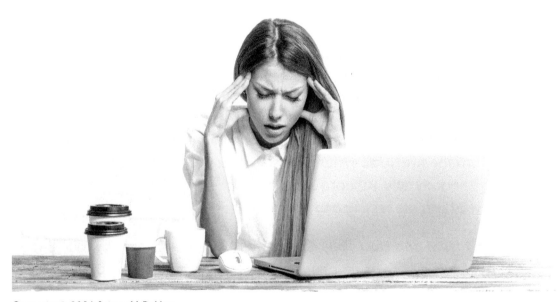

Hans Selye, M.D., our forefather of modern stress studies and world-renowned biologist/ scientist, defined stress in his research as "the non-specific response of the body to any demand made upon it." The intensity of the demand for readjustment or adaptation is what counts. It is possible to predict illness based on the amount of stress in people's lives. What is also significant is how prolonged stress accelerates aging, including that of the skin. Many experts believe that chronic stress releases various hormones such as cortisol and adrenaline and other inflammatory factors. When these substances are produced in excessive amounts over long periods of time, the body's health is seriously compromised producing grave internal chemical changes—by triggering epigenetic tagging, which genes get expressed and which ones stay silent.

Dr. Selye distinguished and coined the term "eustress" for positive stress which is necessary for growth and maintaining optimal health. If stress exceeded the 'healthy' range, it was termed "distress" or negative stress causing dysfunction. The stress that concerns us the most is the damaging "distress" that accumulates in our systems. It leads to disruptions in the body's normal electrical communication systems destroying coherence and producing incoherence which in turn, causes more stress. Dr. Selye maintained in his publications that the most damaging stressors are mental-emotional ones: mental tensions, frustrations, insecurity and aimlessness. Many other researchers are pointing to the same stressors.

Dr. Carolyn DeMarco points out in her book 'Take Charge of Your Body' how women today are facing unique stresses and challenges. The biological changes (that women experience) from their first period, pregnancy to menopause all have their unique life changes and hormonal upheavals. Along with this are the family, money and work stresses that women in particular are managing—when both partners are working, women find themselves still carrying on the traditional marital roles. Women are still responsible in looking after their home and children, doing overtime at work, taking care of meals, finances, volunteering in the community or at school and keeping their husbands happy. Women are often chronically stressed causing serious immune system dysfunctions often due to their never ending list of daily tasks.

Statistics show that women have a higher risk factor for many chronic illnesses, auto immune diseases like lupus, multiple sclerosis and rheumatoid arthritis—plus fibromyalgia, osteoporosis, cancer and even heart disease. Negative stress increases cortisol, "the stress hormone," which in turn causes a negative immune factor Interleukin-6 (IL-6) to be secreted.

Vanderhaeghe & Boucic (1999) stated in their writings that high levels of IL-6 are associated with auto immune conditions (lupus, rheumatoid arthritis, MS), inflammatory diseases and allergies. IL-6 also causes calcium to be pulled from the bones into the blood, aggravating to the osteoporosis condition.

Women have also been found to be shallow breathers, which results in poor oxygenation of the blood, decreasing immunity and impacts the skin (broken capillaries, redness, skin sensitivity). According to Vanderhaeghe, **stress is at the root of women's health issues.**

Dr. DeMarco explains that in almost two thirds of Canadian families, both partners work outside the home. A family today must work 65 to 80 hours a week to maintain the same income that a single breadwinner could obtain from 45 hours of work in the 1970s (DeMarco 1997). DeMarco points out that from a 1992 national mental health survey in Canada, 50 percent of those surveyed felt really stressed three times a week and really depressed at least once a month. I believe that we are seeing more and more women worldwide performing the "super woman roles." As the old cliché states—Woman's work is never done!

STRESS RELATED SKIN PROBLEMS AND ACCELERATED AGING OF THE SKIN

In one study, on the skin's response to stress, the researchers found that stress appears to decrease the skin's ability to function properly and fight disease. Researchers studied 27 students at the University of California, San Francisco, who all had healthy skin. The students were measured on three separate occasions over 8 weeks in 1999. The researchers found that during times of high stress with exams, the skin's ability to recover to normal function (by applying and then stripping sticky tape to aggravate the skin) was decreased. The researchers concluded that they have found a direct link between stress and a decline in the ability of the skin to resume to its normal functions after a disruption. This places stressed-out individuals at a greater risk for developing common skin diseases (e.g. Psoriasis, eczema).

The implications of this study for women are far reaching, as research shows, women are highly stressed out individuals. A scientist by the name of Professor Frances Champagne of Columbia University has been investigating the interplay of epigenetics, linking one's genes and one's environment during the critical process of development.

Dr. Champagne along with her research team examines developmental plasticity in response to environmental experiences. Dr. Champagne uses rodent models to study epigenetics, neurobiology and behavior with a particular interest in the impact of early life experiences on behavior—that is, the neural mechanisms associated with these environmentally mediated effects and the epigenetic changes that allow these effects to persist within and across generations.

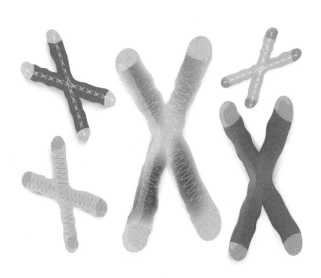

In one of her studies, she focused on whether early childhood conditions can predict coping skills in adults. She found that rat pups whose mothers showed more affection in the first weeks of their lives were far better at coping with stress later on. She points out that similar patterns appear for other species as well- including what happens during abuse. There is evidence that abuse leaves lasting epigenetic changes in primates as well as in human brains (Dr. Champagne).

In recent years, Dr. Elizabeth Blackburn, a molecular biologist and her colleagues have been investigating the effect of stress on telomerase and telomeres. Dr. Blackburn won a Nobel Prize for her work in discovering that stress breaks the genetic strands known as Telomeres. When your telomeres break down so does every part of your body, but especially the skin (See section below on Telomere shrinkage).

Other studies are showing that chronic psychological stress may accelerate aging at the cellular level. One other such study: Intimate partner violence was found to shorten telomere length in formerly abused women versus never abused women, possibly causing poorer overall health and greater morbidity in abused women. This research along with what Dr. Champagne's research showed on the epigenetic changes from abuse is certainly revealing in the aging process.

Researchers are pointing the way that cells are listening in to our thoughts and behaving accordingly. So what kind of thoughts are you entertaining?

Emotions, Chronic Stress and Rate of Telomere Shortening are being shown to age us more than we have realized. Professor, Elissa Epel, UCSF, department of psychiatry asks: **Are Our Cells Listening to Us?** She and her colleagues conducted studies with chronic stress caregivers and monitored their telomeres over a decade. What they found was quite interesting yet not surprising, from what the other studies have shown: **all these caregivers had shortened telomeres!**

> Researchers are pointing the way that cells are listening in to our thoughts and behaving accordingly.

6. TOXIC EMOTIONS—AGES SKIN

"We, ourselves, are what we think. . . . that every fluctuation in thought—in consciousness produces a corresponding change in the body" (Raichur/Cohn, 1997). As pointed out earlier, one of the fundamental causes of imbalance to the body-mind system, which produces hormonal changes and shows up on the skin, is **STRESS!**

Psychoneuroimmunology is now identifying what the ancients knew; how the mind can make us old and sick or also keep us young and well. As Dr. Chopra points out in ***Grow Younger, Live Longer***, *"Agitation in the body and mind creates disease and accelerates aging"* (p 42). We create our body with our thoughts and feelings. It's our perception of stress and how we respond to our perceived stressors.

Mental Health and Your Skin

But there's more that is showing it's not just stress that causes skin problems; anxiety, depression and other psychological conditions do, too. A new field in dermatology has emerged called psycho-dermatology, that the American Psychological Association (APA) says is aimed to understand the relationship between our mental health and skin.

What is interesting is how the new research in this field is suggesting what Ayurvedic traditions have been saying for thousands of years. If you have a skin condition like—acne, rosacea, psoriasis, eczema, whatever it may be—and nothing seems to be working, it might be a psychological issue. "The skin is the most noticeable part of our body that could be impacted by psychological factors, yet very few psychologists are studying it," Kristina G. Gorbatenko-Roth, a psychology professor at the University of Wisconsin-Stout, told the APA. *"It's classic health psychology, just in a different area."*

These new understandings that embrace the holistic viewpoint in skin and health care is certainly coming to light. In the near future, we may see more doctors recommending a daily dose of meditation or mindfulness exercises more readily than a topical cream.

7. MITOCHONDRIAL DYSFUNCTION

Mitochondrial dysfunction is considered a hallmark of aging and considered to be more accurate than the Free radical theory. It has become a spotlight in the research on aging. Mitochondria are found in every cell of the human body except red blood cells and convert the energy of food molecules into the ATP that powers most cell functions as well as the purging of toxic debris.

A Harvard Professor of Genetics David Sinclair, the principal researcher on a mitochondrial study, theorized that aging occurs because the communication between the mitochondria and the nucleus inside our cells breaks down as we get older. Dr. Sinclair's results have given scientific evidence that he is correct.

Mitochondria are responsible for creating more than 90% of the energy needed by the body to sustain life and support growth. When they fail, less and less energy is generated within the cell. Cell injury and even cell death follow.

Since the mitochondria are responsible for processing oxygen and converting substances from the foods we eat into energy for essential cellular functions, it has been found that impairment of mitochondrial function and/or increased oxidative damage leads to the onset of many defects for adults. These include Type 2 diabetes, Parkinson's disease, skeletal muscle aging, atherosclerotic heart disease, stroke, Alzheimer's disease, and cancer. Many medicines can also injure the mitochondria. This new research by Sinclair's landmark 2013 study, shows that aging can be slowed down. And that the key to slowing down aging, or even reversing it, is in a molecule called **Nicotinamide Adeine Dinucleotide**, or NAD+. Sinclair discovered a way to nutritionally provide for NAD+.

NAD+ is an essential metabolite in all human cells and plays a key role in cellular metabolism and energy production. It is vital for mitochondrial health. As we age, we lose up to 50% of our NAD+, causing our cells to produce less and less energy.

These results are the typical **aging symptoms**—grey hair, wrinkles, decreased energy... followed later by memory loss, disease and death. Dr. Sinclair has discovered a dietary precursor to NAD+ which is responsible for facilitating communication between the cell's nucleus (the "brain" of the cell) and mitochondria (the "power plants" of the cell). Other nutrients have also been identified to restore aging mitochondria—which is presented in the antioxidant chapter.

8. TELOMERE SHRINKAGE

Scientists the world over have been studying telomeres and the role they play in human aging or cellular senescence. What they have found has been attributed to the shortening of telomeres of the DNA with each cell cycle.

Cells stay young as long as they are able to repair their own DNA and that is dictated by the telomeres, the proteins at the end of each chromosome. When telomeres become too short, the cells die. American anatomist Leonard Hayflick in 1961 discovered that human cells divide for a limited number of times **in vitro, calling the telomeres** the "molecular clock." or the Hayflick limit.

Inside the nucleus of virtually all of our cells are chromosomes—the 23 pairs of tightly wound strands of DNA—which contain our genes and the cell has many mechanisms to safeguard their well-being. One of these is the telomere, which is located at the tip of these chromosomes like a plastic cap at the end of a shoelace, which keeps chromosomes from fraying and genes from unraveling. Telomeres are important for replication or duplication of the chromosomes during cell division.

But as we age, these tips shorten until eventually they are so short that no further cell division can occur. Eventually they lose their protective power. When that happens, cells either undergo apoptosis (cell suicide), so they can be replaced by healthier cells, or they go into an inactive retirement called senescence unable to divide further and eventually malfunction. Some of these cells even die. While some have likened this to a genetic biological clock, others have described telomeres as a fuse that becomes shorter and shorter, until it sets off a kind of cellular time bomb that wreaks havoc on the cell's internal workings. **The process is behind much of the wear and tear associated with aging.**

Researchers studying Telomeres are showing how important they are to aging. At birth they tend to be around 8,000 base pairs long, around 35 years they are 3,000 base pairs long and by age 65 they can be less than 1,500 base pairs long.

The difference in length is quite significant—and there are a number of factors that make them short. In one study, researchers found that women with chronically ill children had dramatically shorter telomere chains than those of women with low stress children. Emotions and mental states such as anxiety and depression play a huge part in telomere and cellular health. Lifestyle changes can make a difference in both increasing telomere length and protecting existent telomeres from further damage (www.oracvalues.com). Researchers have identified some of these lifestyle changes that can protect telomeres from shortening prematurely include: eating an antioxidant rich diet, reducing stress, increasing positive feelings, exercising, improving your sleep quality and increasing vitamin D production.

Chromosome

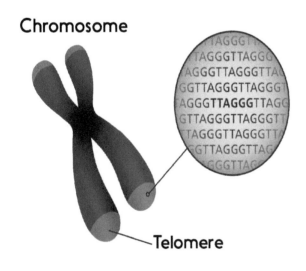

Telomere

Antioxidants are playing a more significant role as they are often credited in providing the necessary nutritional support to help protect normal telomere size and function. According to some recent research, Green tea drinkers have longer telomeres than non-tea drinkers.

The continual challenge for researchers has been to find a way to increase the length of telomeres for different cell types when aging typically shortens them, on average, 1% per year. Scientists have made many advances and have already identified steps you can take right now to take advantage of the Nobel Prize winning discovery of telomeres. **Professor Elizabeth Helen Blackburn**, co-discovered telomerase, the enzyme that replenishes the telomere. For this work, she was awarded the 2009 Nobel Prize in Physiology of Medicine, sharing it with Carol W. Greider and Jack W. Szostak.

They also found that telomeres are very sensitive to the environment and your thoughts. Meditation has been shown to slow cell aging along with consciousness or being fully in the present moment, the mindfulness studies. In another study, people with more tendencies for mind-wandering had shorter telomeres than those who were more present in each moment.

Dr. C. Norman Shealy, neurosurgeon, longevity researcher and founder of the Shealy Pain Clinic points out that science has established that those who live to age 100 have exceptionally long 'telomeres'. The tips of their DNA strands have not been shortened. People who have longer telomeres live longer lives and are less susceptible to some diseases. He points out that: *for the first time in science we have the data from clinical studies whereby telomeres can be regenerated in healthy people.* More discoveries are being made in the area of telomeres and the DNA which is revolutionizing our concepts of life and certainly aging as we have known it.

9. BIOLOGICAL CLOCK

Genetics plays a minor role in how your skin ages, Dr. Perricone, dermatologist and author of **The Wrinkle Cure**, identifies a number of other reasons for the natural aging process. He explains how the skin, overtime, will diminish in its ability to produce necessary oils and functions. Some of these include:

- Dryness of the skin due to reduced oil gland production after age 30.
- Reduced ability of skin to ward off sun damage.
- Sagging and thinning of the skin to occur at the ages 40–50 due to the loss of the fat layer.
- Skin firmness diminishes which results in collagen and elastin reduction, immune response diminishes along with the ability to repair damage.

Thus the road to help with this 'biological clock' ticking away is to support our body-mind even more so with the choices we make regarding our food, our nutrients, exercise or body-movements, our thoughts, our emotions and how we handle stressors. Suzanne Somers says it wisely in **Bombshell**: *"We are in control of how well we age."*

10. HIGH TECH GADGETS AGING US AND MAKING US SICK

The Electromagnetic pollution Era: Electromagnetic pollution that emanates from all our high tech gadgets—cell phones and even our cars—emit electromagnetic radiation that can penetrate and affect us, seriously compromising our health and disturbing our environments.

We are exposed to **200,000,000 times** more EM fields in our environment today than our ancestors. This is WAY more than our circuits can handle.

There are more studies that exist today showing the adverse effects of EMF's (electromagnetic fields) than there are studies showing the risks for cancer by smokers. Scientists have conducted research linking EM radiation to serious diseases like cancer, Alzheimer's disease, Parkinson's disease and others.

Research now links long-term exposure to electromagnetic fields (EMFs) with chronic health issues, from stress and fatigue to cancer. Overwhelming numbers of scientists now agree that EMFs are carcinogens. **But, like any massive public health threat, it may be years before the talk stops and the action starts. In the meantime, people are getting sick.** EMFs (also called Electro-Smog) are invisible, silent and ubiquitous.

In May 2006, the London Observer reported the growing concern about what it called the 'invisible smog' that has been created by the 'electricity that powers our civilization'. Scientific evidence showed that this was:

- giving children cancer
- causing miscarriages
- suicides
- making some people allergic to 'modern life'

EMF is classified as a Group 2B carcinogen under standards established by the World Health Organization's Agency for Cancer Research. The chemicals DDT and lead are also Group 2B carcinogens (Source: National Institute for Environmental Health Sciences).

Studies have shown that people who are exposed to magnetic fields higher than 2.5 mG have an increased risk of cancer and other diseases. Millions of computers in use in the workplace emit magnetic fields higher than 3 mG. Electromagnetic fields interfere with the balance and harmony of the body's electromagnetic field and its electrical communication systems through something called 'entrainment.'

Dr. Devra Davis one of the most well-respected and credentialed researchers warns that **cell phone radiation is as dangerous as carcinogenic pesticides—which**

have been banned world-wide—yet, even though cell phones are classified by the International Agency

for Research on Cancer as a Class 2B carcinogen, they are still in common use. Just look around you and you'll see that cell phones with their variations of I-phones, androids etc. have increased in usage and has created another peculiarity called "Tech-neck wrinkles" (See below for more description).

In June 2012, a Toronto hospital was the first to formally recognize symptoms from wireless radiation. Women's College Hospital urged family doctors to learn to detect the symptoms of wireless radiation exposure. They include **disrupted sleep, headaches, nausea, dizziness, heart palpitations, memory problems and skin rashes. This condition is being labelled Electro-magnetic Hyper-sensitivity, or "EMS."**

Skin rashes and blotchy skin is more common from EMF WIFI exposure than most realize. One of my clients who was unable to resolve a very serious skin disorder, was finally able to receive relief and healing when the WIFI was switched off in her home.

Other studies have examined the possible effects of 60-Hz electromagnetic field exposure on the pineal gland function in humans. The findings have been quite revealing: they show that indeed EMF's even **extremely low frequency electric or magnetic fields can affect pineal gland function. (***Vibrational Cleaning***)** In my own work with the GDV Kirlian camera, I consistently noticed bio-field changes—or interruptions, sometimes huge gaps would appear above and around the head area. Since the pineal gland is our anti-aging gland, this type of disruption obviously would only accelerate the aging process.

11. NEW 'TECH-NECK' WRINKLES

Now this is definitely, a 21st century, cyberspace phenomenon that is attracting more attention. Dermatologists have given this name `tech-neck` wrinkles to those that are glued to their smart phones. Dermatologists are blaming smart phones and tablets for causing sagging skin and wrinkles in younger generations, including a wrinkling condition dubbed "tech neck". They say that this is mostly found in people aged **18 to 39** who own an average of three devices.

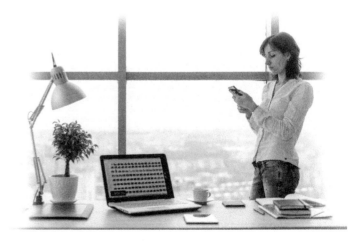

Is this you? Tech neck refers to a specific crease just above the collar bone that is caused by repeated bending of the neck that is, **looking down and staring at your smart phone and tablet screens 150 times a day thereby causing droopy jowls, saggy skin and crinkly clavicles.**

Dr Christopher Rowland Payne, Consultant Dermatologist at The London Clinic, said in an interview that: "The problem of wrinkles and sagging of the jowls and neck used to begin in late middle age but, in the last 10 years, because of 'tech-neck', it has become a problem for a generation of younger women." Now **dermatologists are addressing this new phenomenon with new potions and lotions! I have addressed it too but with natural skin tighteners in Chapter 13.**

DON'T BLAME YOUR GENES—IT'S YOUR ENVIRONMENT!

According to Br. Bruce Lipton, researcher, author, quantum biologist, he says that your environment, your thoughts dictate the expression of your DNA.

Genetics account for only 25 to 35 percent of how fast you age-the rest is determined by your choices, your attitude, your beliefs, your environment and your metabolism.

SUMMARY OF AGING ACCELERATORS

- Telomeres shortening—the loss of telomeres
- Sun damage
- Smart phone/tablet usage—`tech-neck`
- Cigarette smoke (including second hand)—Free Radical Damage
- Coffee, sugar, alcohol—junk food
- Poor Digestion—lack of enzymes & Probiotics
- Hormonal fluctuations—imbalances
- Chemicals, pollutants—environmental exposures
- Polluted indoor environments—household cleaners
- Habitual facial expressions
- Abrasive soaps and chemical carcinogens in cosmetics
- Lack of proper skin care
- Toxic emotions/attitudes
- Toxic, stressed liver
- Poor nutrition (especially vitamins A, C and E)
- Poor Fatty Acid absorption or imbalance
- Mitochondrial dysfunction
- Sleep Deprivation or poor sleep
- Beliefs and perceptions of aging
- Stress (Psychological and Emotional) Levels
- Adrenal Burn-Out
- Electromagnetic Pollution

CHAPTER 5

WHY ESSENTIAL OILS?

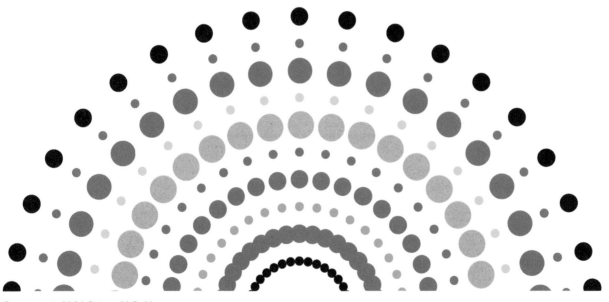

"Every flower is a soul blossoming in nature."
GERARD DE NERVAL

"Aromatherapy carries a message of life and hope for tens of millions and perhaps hundreds of millions of people."
DANIEL PONOÉL

ANCIENT WAYS

Essential oils have been around for thousands of years. In fact, therapeutic, spiritual and cosmetic uses of aromatic oils have at least a 6,000-year history. The ancient Egyptians used them in the embalming process as well as for health, healing and cosmetic fragrances. Beauty and cosmetics were of prime importance to Egyptians, both in their daily life and for the afterlife. They took their personal hygiene seriously, as illustrated by the earliest recorded recipe of a body deodorant found in the Papyrus Ebers of 1500 BC (Worwood 1990). Perhaps the Egyptians were the first cosmetic chemists as they used their talents to embalm and preserve the flesh of their Pharaohs to treating the skin of their living.

The first archaeological evidence of cosmetics that was used in Ancient Egypt dates back to 4000 B.C. The ancient Egyptians regarded beauty as a sign of holiness. They regarded cosmetics as having magical powers and thus used them as an integral part of their daily lives. Egyptians used cosmetics regardless of sex and social status for aesthetic, religious and therapeutic reasons.

Oils and unguents were rubbed into the skin to protect it from the hot air. Everything the ancient Egyptians used had a spiritual aspect to it. Because cosmetics were regarded as being important for their magical and religious purposes in the after world, cosmetics were among the offerings left in tombs. Cosmetic palettes were found buried with the deceased as grave goods. Those who could afford it had seven creams and two kinds of rouge put into their tombs when they died.

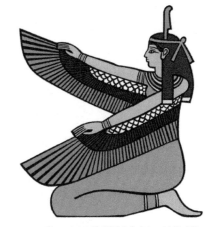

Records show that Mineral makeup was used by the Egyptian women. They applied a bright green paste of copper minerals to their faces to provide color. They used kohl to line their eyes, because they believed it protected them from the harmful sun rays. They also wore green eyeliner made from crushed malachite stone. The sculptures of the Egyptian women show painted eyes. Perfumes of all sorts were used on the body and their clothes, and homes were made fragrant with various essential oils, especially myrrh oil.

Ancient Greeks, Romans and Egyptians used cosmetics made out of mercury, white lead, frankincense and myrrh.

Then, in the tenth century, the famous Arabian physician Avicenna wrote over a hundred books, the first of which was an entire book on the beneficial effects of the rose. The earliest scriptures of the Hindu religion, the Vedas, codify several hundred perfumes and aromatic products. This knowledge was maintained for at least 6,000 years through Indian Ayurvedic medicine which advocated aromatic massage as its principal practice and still does today.

Aromatic oils were the key ingredients in the earliest cosmetics. Ancient Egyptians lavished in aromatic baths and anointed their bodies to keep their skin healthy and youthful. The Egyptians were also known to design personal perfumes to elicit various emotions and inspire thoughts. Peter and Kate Damian point out in ***Aromatherapy, Scent and Psyche*** how the Egyptians also used fragrances to honor, appease and solicit favors from the gods. Eventually, they used scents for nearly every purpose, from battle to spiritual ecstasy. In about 1500 BC, Queen Hatshepsut was instrumental in advancing the use of cosmetics and perfumes amongst her subjects. She also revered the myrrh tree to such an extent that she had them transplanted throughout various areas in Egypt. The Greeks expanded the use of aromatherapy in aesthetic pursuits of beauty and romance. They had a very high opinion of aromatics, attributing sweet smells to the divine. They introduced the art of perfumery to the Romans.

Cleopatra was extravagant in her use of roses and other aromatics, and especially to seduce Mark Antony. The Greeks and Romans lavished in oils with their frequent baths and massages. The Romans would run rose water via canals throughout their gardens and palaces (there were over a thousand scented watering pools in the city) where bathers could be anointed and massaged with aromatic oils. Well-preserved essential oils were found in alabaster jars in King Tut's tomb in 1992. Since then European scientists have rediscovered the many healing properties of essential oils.

WHAT ARE ESSENTIAL OILS?

Essential oils are distilled from plants as a subtle volatile liquid (they evaporate readily when exposed to air). Essential oils are the life force, the regenerating and oxygenating immune

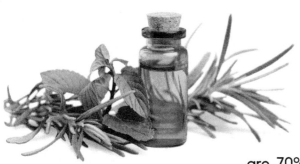

defense properties of plants. Essential oils also have hormone-like properties. They are extremely concentrated and are often referred to as the heart, soul or spirit of aromatic plants. They are the source of all fragrance in plant life.

Raichur/Cohn reports in her book that essential oils are 70% to 80% more concentrated than herbal powders. They have a very unique lipid structure including oxygenating molecules that gives them the ability to penetrate cell membranes, and transport oxygen and nutrients inside each cell of the body within only 21 minutes of their application and, in some cases, within seconds. This is in sharp contrast to the average of 13 to 24 hours for the therapeutic constituents of dried herbs to reach the cells.

Essential oils are one of the highest known sources of antioxidants that can prevent free radical damage (more on this in Chapter 8).

Cosmetic Benefits of Essential Oils

1. They stimulate skin cells into reproducing at a quicker rate thus reducing the time lag between new skin growth and elimination of old cells. This helps to reverse the process of aging.

2. Penetrates and moisturizes deep layer in the skin.

3. Helps to heal skin damaged by sun, burns and wrinkles.

4. Prevents the congestion of toxins and expedites the elimination of toxic debris thereby improving lymphatic flow.

5. Destroys infectious agents, re. acne and skin infections.

6. Helps to reduce puffiness and inflammation.

7. Helps to relieve the stress and tension that so often leads directly to aging skin.

8. Supports the regulation of over or underactive oil glands.

9. Contains plant hormones.

10. Nutrients and proteins contained in the essential oils work as a restorative building block to keeping collagen and elastin in good condition.

Furthermore, the beauty in using essential oils, as pointed out by Dr. David Stewart, Ph.D., in his book 'Healing Oils of the Bible' is that "they don't have negative side effects like the synthetic drugs and chemicals of modern pharmacology." They are non-toxic, harmless to human tissue and promote healing.

Essential oils work on many different levels: Physically, emotionally, psychologically and spiritually. **They produce effects 60% to 75% stronger** than herbs taken whole. (Raichur/Cohn).

They also work through the sense of smell (most sensitive of the five senses) and through the skin. Your skin can absorb the molecules of essential oils easily by traveling through the pores, hair follicles and the intercellular fluid surrounding the skin cells. They travel into your blood stream, reaching the internal organs and lymphatic system. Essential oils are transdermal and reach any part of your body within minutes. For example, place an oil such as Clove or Peppermint on the soles of your feet and you can taste the oil on your tongue in less than a minute.

In the *Fragrant Pharmacy* by Valerie Ann Worwood and *Aromatherapy for Dummies* by Kathi Keville, both authors point out the many virtues of what essential oils do cosmetically for the skin which is summarized in the following chart.

Essential oils have a unique and superior advantage over other substances because of their capacity to advance cellular renewal by increasing circulation, hydration and waste removal. Essential oils have a natural regulatory homeostatic function as they can invigorate or stabilize internal organs. Essential oils contain **natural antibacterial, antiseptic, anti-fungal and preservative properties**. Many essential oils have *cell-regenerating properties, helping to make the skin smooth* and youthful. Essential oils boost immunity, reduce stress, calm nerves, balance moods—essential oils are definitely an ally to have in caring for your body, face, mind and spirit.

Researchers have shown that people who surround themselves with pleasant scents enjoy higher self esteem and well-being. Whatever you choose to do, essential oils offer you a wealth of benefits including emotional balance. You cannot overdo aromatherapy, or do it wrong; just be creative in pampering yourself. This book would not be complete without briefly describing the other great well-known virtue of essential oils—the power of smell or the olfactory system!

"Look in the perfumes of flowers and of nature
for peace of mind and joy of life."
WANG WEI, 8TH CENTURY AD

EMOTIONS AND AROMAS: THE NOSE KNOWS

The human olfactory system—sense of smell—is our most ancient and powerful root of our emotional life. (Goleman, 1997) Research has shown that aromas stimulate the brain within one to three seconds. As aromatic molecules are inhaled, olfactory membranes lined with receptor cells capture them.

Limbic system of the brain

Olfactory bulb

Nasal cavity

Aromatic substances

Olfactory neurons

There are 800 million nerve endings for processing and detecting odors. Each fragrance molecule fits itself into specific receptor cells, like a puzzle piece. The stimulation created by the odor causes the receptors to trigger electrical impulses to the olfactory bulb deep into 'the "old" brain or limbic system (the electrical switchboard for the brain) within milliseconds, bypassing the thalamus..

The olfactory bulb transmits the information to the gustatory center (taste sensations), the amygdala (where emotional memories are stored) and other parts of the brain that control heart rate, blood pressure, breathing, memory, stress levels and hormone balance. Because of this, the essential oils have profound physiological and psychological effects. (Young, 2003)

Out of the five senses, smell is the only one that is directly linked to the limbic lobe of the brain; our emotional center. Emotions such as anger, depression, fear and joy emanate from this region. Special aromas can evoke memories and emotions before we are even consciously aware of them. Essential oils, through their fragrance, can directly stimulate both the limbic lobe and the hypothalamus—affecting the production of hormones. In this way, essential oils have a most powerful effect on the body and mind.

Dr. C. Pert in **Molecules of Emotion** (1997) describes how the sense of smell is only one synapse away from the nose to the amygdala. This is the area in the brain which directly routes incoming sensory information in all forms to the higher centers of association in the cortex. This is why odors are so strong and memorable—giving them a unique capacity to evoke emotions. Scientists have learned that oil fragrances may be one of the fastest ways to achieve body-mind changes that affect mood, wakefulness, anxiety, stress levels, etc. Findings show that oils such as orange, jasmine and rose have a tranquilizing effect and work by altering brain waves into a rhythm that produces calmness and a sense of well-being.

Stimulating oils, like **basil, black pepper, rosemary and cardamom** work by producing a **heightened energy response**. A study conducted by Professor Jacob at Cardiff University in England analyzed the effect of **ylang ylang and rosemary** essential oils on brain wave activity using an electroencephalograph (EEF). *Ylang Ylang* produced dramatic rises in alpha wave amplitude—a sign of relaxation. *Rosemary* essential oil resulted in a decrease in alpha wave amplitude—**a sign of alertness!**

Modern scientists who are studying the psycho physiological and behavioral effects of aromas can be thankful to Dr. Gattefossé who renewed the use of essential oils by accident. In 1910, Dr. Gattefossé French cosmetic chemist was set aflame following a laboratory explosion. After extinguishing the flames, he found that both his hands were covered in "rapidly developing gas gangrene." He plunged his hands and arms into a vat of **lavender oil** thinking it was water. The **lavender oil** stopped the gasification of the tissue with just one rinse. When the wound healed within hours with no infection or scarring, this prompted Dr. Gattefossé to intensify his research on essential oils (Young, 2003). He has been credited with the coining of the term "**aromatherapy**." Cosmetic aromatherapy takes advantage of the essential oils' capacity to balance our mind, emotions and spirit. Dr. Julian Whitaker says it so simply, "that sometimes the answer to stress may be right under your nose" (1997:219).

By using scents on your face, the essential oils not only feed/nurture/rejuvenate your skin, but also balance your mind, body and emotions. It's such a powerful and common "scents" thing to do!

Fragrances from chemical scents are non-sense to use!

It is not worth dying for "good looks" or "fragrant synthetic smells!"

Rather, it makes common "scents" to use Mother Nature's most sacred, natural plant aromas. The question is where do we obtain them?

ESSENTIAL OILS HAVE A DIRECT IMPACT ON:

- **Memory**: Links to the same part of the brain that links the experience with the aroma
- **Emotional response**: Molecules trigger nerve impulses to the specific brain region- amygdala—associated with certain emotions.
- **Body response**: Impacts the autonomic system and the subconscious thus releasing hormonal production and hormonal circulation.

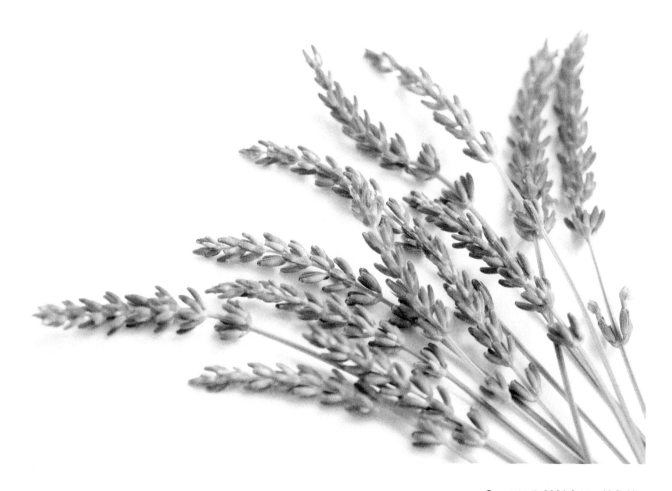

THE IMPORTANCE OF QUALITY

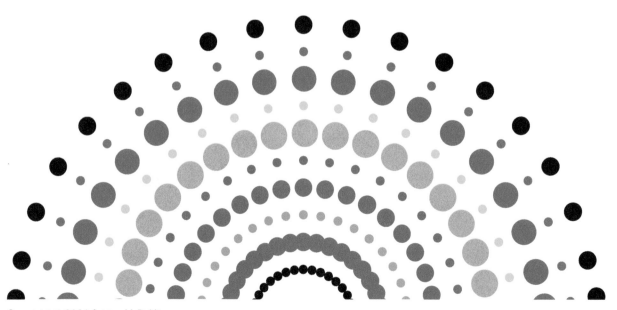

"The whole of an essential oil is greater than the sum of its parts, especially since we don't know what all those parts are."
DAMIANS, 1995

NOT ALL OILS ARE CREATED EQUAL

Many of the authors referred to in this book advocate the use of pure organic plant extracts. There is a difference between organic (natural) and synthetic oils. Not any essential oil will do. An organic and natural essential oil contains at least several hundred components that work **synergistically**, making the oils unique, safe and effective. For example, natural rose oil may have as many as **2,000 components** whereas synthetic rose oil may have only 50 components. The combination of constituents as found in an essential oil and created by Mother Nature is more effective than an isolated constituent.

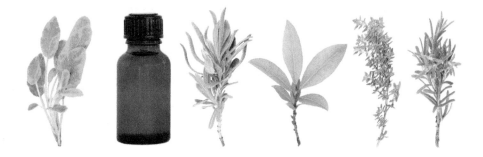

The essential oils are highly concentrated substances with strong electromagnetic, biological and chemical activities that work with the body's subtle intelligence and wisdom. Synthetic, adulterated or tainted oils put a person at a greater risk to experience symptoms of toxicity, allergies, sensitivities and irritation. These lifeless pseudo-aromatic chemicals (the Damians like to call them "aroma-drugs") become toxic waste in the body, causing a host of symptoms as discussed earlier in Chapter 1. People who have sensitivities and allergies to commercial, synthetic fragrances are often not reactive to pure, high quality essential oils. This was certainly the case for me—**Synthetic essences can never replace the holistic action and intelligence of Mother Nature's own creation—essential oils.**

Many of the oils on the market today are synthetic, inexpensive oils, perfume quality, adulterated, over processed, chemical-laden and denatured or added mimicker compounds. After all, 98% of essential oils are used in the perfume and cosmetic industry, leaving only 2% produced as therapeutic or genuine grade oils. Which ones are the true genuine/therapeutic grade oils? How will you know? What are some of the facts that will help you?

MORE ON WHY I CHOSE YOUNG LIVING?

I have outlined earlier in the Preface, my personal search and discovery with Young Living Essential Oils. **The quality of an oil is everything**. One of the key factors in producing a genuine/ therapeutic-grade quality essential oil is in preserving the delicate aromatic compounds within the essential oils which means—no synthetic chemical or solvent is to be used in it. These fragile aromatic compounds are easily destroyed by high temperature and high pressure. Contact with chemically reactive metals such as copper or aluminum during distillation also destroy these fragile aromatic compounds in the oils. It becomes imperative (in order to ensure a Genuine/therapeutic-grade essential oil) that all essential oils are distilled in stainless steel cooking chambers at low pressure and low temperature.

The other key factor to ensure a high quality oil is in having organically grown botanicals. The plants and herbs need to be free of herbicides, pesticides and chemical fertilizers. These toxic agrichemicals can react with the essential oil during distillation producing toxic compounds.

The purity of essential oils is also determined by a number of other conditions based on **soil quality, location, climate, altitude, growing and harvesting methods, distillation process, organic farming practices and quality of seed selection.**

THE FIELDS—WHERE BEAUTY BEGINS

On the farmland in Idaho and Utah lie the spectacular organic herb gardens that are owned by Young Living. On the next page, the photo is a lavender field in full bloom. From these fragrant flowers, the oil of lavender is gently distilled, preserving its natural soothing and healing qualities, so valuable in maintaining one's health, beauty and youthful appearance.

Young Living's statement to quality: "We select and cultivate only the species of herbs that will produce the most active and widest array of constituents."

"We grow herbs on land uncontaminated by pesticides, herbicides. . . . We irrigate with pure mountain water. . . . And maintain the soil with enzymes and trace minerals. The herbs

are distilled fresh on the farm . . . we distill our own essential oils under low pressure and low temperature to preserve the healing constituents." (D. Gary Young).

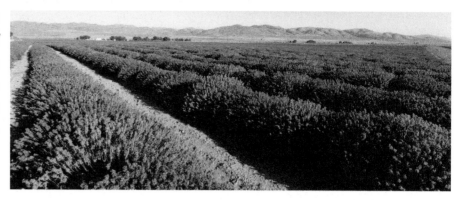

HOW DO YOU THE CONSUMER KNOW IF THE ESSENTIAL OILS ARE TOP QUALITY?

A set of standards has been established in Europe that qualifies a therapeutic-grade oil. These standards are known as AFNOR (Association French Normalization Organization Regulation) or ISO certification (International Standards Organization—which has set the international standards for therapeutic-grade essential oils adopted from AFNOR). The AFNOR or ISO certification has been the most reliable indicators of essential oil quality. But there are other standards that are important to investigate as well.

Natural beauty and vibrancy starts from the herbs, which embody the essential oils – the heart and spirit of aromatic plants. The vital energy, beauty and life force of the plant is brought directly to your skin by using (this wonderful treasure) essential oils.

AFNOR was developed by a team led by government-certified botanical chemist, Hervé Casabianca, Ph.D. while working with several analytical laboratories throughout France. Dr. Casabianca qualifies an oil as therapeutic when the primary constituents within an essential oil occur in certain percentages. He has collaborated his work with other scientists, that include the French government certified laboratory called Central Service Analysis Laboratory.

To give you an example, lavender oil is frequently produced from hybrids, claiming to be genuine oil. The AFNOR standard for true lavender (Lavandula angustifolia) dictates what the range from constituents should be, (i.e., linalool from 25 to 38%, linalyl acetate from 25 to 34%) to be therapeutic grade. Tasmania produces a lavandin that mimics the chemistry of true lavender. The only way to determine if the oil is authentic is to analyze the chemical fingerprint using high-resolution gas chromatography and compare it with AFNOR standard for genuine lavender. (Young 2003).

Almost all labs in the U.S. are ill-equipped to analyze natural chemicals in essential oils as their equipment is designed to analyze synthetic chemicals and marker compounds in vitamins and minerals. There is no agency in the world to regulate and certify therapeutic-grade essential oils.

The only means, at present, is if it meets AFNOR or ISO standards. So far, only two companies use the proper machinery and test standards for AFNOR essential oil analysis—Flora Research and Young Living Essential Oils.

Young Living takes extraordinary steps to their growing, harvesting and distilling of the plants. Plants are distilled in small batches for extended periods at low pressure and low heat in stainless steel vertical steam distillers developed by D. Gary Young (which minimizes chemical alterations from reactive metals). No solvents or synthetic chemicals of any kind are used.

Timing and pressure in distillation are extremely important; e.g. Cypress requires 24 hours at 245 degrees F and 5 pounds of pressure to extract all of its active ingredients. Lessening the time by 2 hours will result in destroying 18 to 20 of the oil's constituents. Most operations distill Cypress for only 1 hour and 15 minutes—you can imagine the quality of the oil.

Daniel Penoél, M.D., a leader, practitioner and researcher of 25 years in the use of essential oils and author of **Natural Home Health Care Using Essential Oils** says, as his motto, *"I would rather have a drop of genuine essential oils than a 55-gallon drum of junk product."* He points out how quality essential oils are expensive to produce but they are worth it. He also points out in his introductory letter in the "An Introduction to Young Living Essential Oils" booklet how many companies have jumped onto the aromatic bandwagon for commercial reasons—selling products for recreational 'fragrancing.' This usually means emphasis is placed on **decreasing quality for quantity**. Dr. Penoél states that this is not the case with Young Living. *"Instead Young Living's founder and president, Gary Young, has created a means for producing therapeutic-grade essential oils—"oils of the very highest quality"—on a very large scale.*

"I found them [the Young Living oils] to be top quality, definitely deserving of the term 'therapeutic grade.'" Dr. Penoél continues to say in his **Natural Home** book, *"I congratulate Gary for his incredible agricultural and distillation accomplishments in Utah and Idaho. This is precisely my picture of 'healing the planet' and creating a vast, beautiful fragrant garden"* (1998, p 8).

The quality of Young Living's pure and potent essential oils has established credibility with eminent scientists and medical professionals worldwide, who continue to research and validate the effectiveness of these timeless natural wonders. The following comparison outlines the significant differences of Genuine (bio-dynamic-organic) vs. Synthetic — Adulterated oils.

GENUINE THERAPEUTIC-GRADE OILS	SYNTHETIC ADULTERATED-GRADE OILS
• The pure essence of roots, leaves and flowers are carefully distilled from wild or organically grown plants. The result is unadulterated essential oils that exhibit powerful effects on the body and the mind.	• The aroma may be mingled with chemical pesticides, fungicides or fertilizers. Additives may be used to dilute the oil or the scent may result from artificial substances created in the laboratory.
• Pure oils obtained from correctly identified plant species, offering naturally occurring, therapeutic-grade constituents.	• An oil modified with synthetic chemical components to obtain the desired aroma, without the therapeutic-grade constituents.
• Pure mountain water is used for the distillation process, keeping the oils free of additives.	• Water for distillation may be treated with chlorine, fluorine and a lot of other chemicals that may mix with oils.
• A proprietary stainless steel distillation process using low temperatures and pressure to preserve all plant properties and constituents.	• High pressure, high heat, metal distilleries react chemically with the oils and damage beneficial constituents.
• Using long, slow distillation time to capture the pure essence of the plant and preserve the quality of the essential oils.	• Quick distillation processes damage the oils and decrease its overall quality.
• The process provides authentic, pure, therapeutic-grade essential oils	• The process results in low-grade, low-quality oils and adulterated mixes.

Young Living Scentsability Brochure

Finding companies that produce organic, genuine/ therapeutic Grade A essential oils can be a challenge. They do exist. There are only a very few high quality companies that adhere to the rigor and commitment for quality. Always ask:

a) Can you eat their oils—are they edible? and better still

b) Can the company's oils be used for Intravenous purposes? or

c) Can they be used for Stem Cell injections?

It is important to know what to look for and what to ask. Every day consumers unknowingly purchase "pseudo-aromatherapy" products from companies who are mass-producing petro-chemical imposters. About 95% of the products sold as aromatherapy is counterfeit (R. Wilson) which offer no therapeutic value whatsoever. Be aware that just because a company may make a claim that their oils are therapeutic it does not mean that they are. So, make sure to ask the above questions.

Roberta Wilson, in her book on aromatherapy, also points out those farmers who grow botanicals all organically help to counter soil erosion, reduce toxic wastes and help the ecosystem. *"Each time you purchase pure essential oils, you cast a vote for natural botanicals that can have immediate and long term effects on your health, well-being and longevity as well as on the health, well-being and future of the planet."*

- Make sure you purchase oils that are derived from organically grown or wild crafted plants (no solvents/no dilution/no adulteration).
- Steam distilled at the correct pressure and low temperatures in non-reactive vessels.
- Bottled in dark or opaque containers.
- Not oily when rubbed between the fingers.
- Non-alcohol smelling.
- Stored at room temperature or cooler and out of direct sunlight.

I strongly agree with her comments. Your purchasing power, your pocketbook makes a statement that helps in supporting environmental sustainable farms! You vote with your money—and you can help Mother Earth immensely in what you buy and support. Young Living's 'Seed to Seal' is certainly a hall-mark in supporting sustainable farming.

NUTRITION AND ANTIOXIDANTS

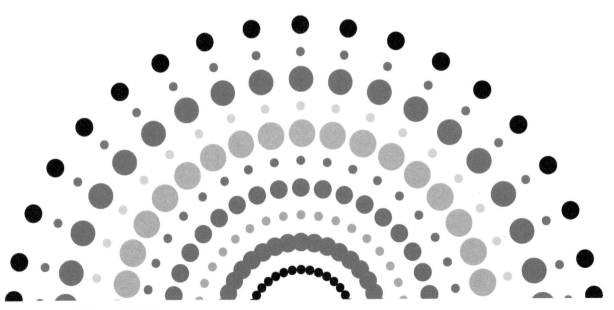

*"Everything has beauty,
but not everyone sees it."*
CONFUCIUS

NUTRITION

Most people are aware that what you eat is reflected on your face. I like to put it simply by saying: "what's that on your fork?" Are you making sure that the foods you're putting on your plate are foods that will give you healthy skin? If you truly want fabulous, glowing, vibrant and younger-looking skin, younger feeling, vibrant body then everything you eat and/or drink becomes critical. In the quest for natural beauty, health and vitality, remember that Mother Nature provides everything you need to encourage and support the healthy functioning of your skin, and your body-mind, but it is up to you to accept her offerings. The less attention you pay to what goes into your mouth, the more problems you may see cropping up as a skin condition. The everyday things you can do to beautify your skin are remarkably similar to what you can do to live longer and healthier—Get regular exercise, sleep enough, have a positive attitude, be in loving thoughts, avoid sun damage and consume clean, organic, healthy foods/water—along with the most important in your to do list:

CLEANSE THE TOXINS!

In order to appreciate the role of proper food intake, nutrition and a healthier lifestyle, I have created and summarized major facial concerns (thanks to M. Rothkranz and M. Kushi) that correspond to internal organs in the chart on the following pages (Also see Appendix E).

FACIAL SIGNS SPEAK

FACIAL CONCERN	INTERNAL PROBLEMATIC CONCERN
Middle Forehead lines	Small Intestines & nervous system Circulation
Deep creases in forehead & between eyes	Liver & large intestines
Forehead Corners (above eyebrows) lines	Bladder, Kidneys
Eyebrows	Bladder, Kidneys
Lighter in color	Weak Kidneys
Longer eyebrows	Healthier
Eyes —area around eyes	Kidneys: Can also be indicative of too much animal protein/cooked fats/drugs/ medications
Swelling, sagging or dark circles	Kidneys are struggling (water issues plus also protein, starches, sugar, toxins and emotional issues)
Dark Circles	Kidneys and adrenals are exhausted
Tired eyes	Liver depletion
Bulging eyes	Thyroid problems (usually hyperactive)
Eye bags	Kidneys are swollen: body is tired, overloaded, too much liquid
	Mucus, fat accumulation clogging bladder, or urethra, ovaries, uterus, prostate & testicles
Frown lines between eyebrows	Liver—also includes emotions like anger
Crow`s Feet—wrinkles	Liver cleanse is needed
Outside of eye bags	Adrenals

FACIAL CONCERN	INTERNAL PROBLEMATIC CONCERN
Nose—(red or swollen)	Heart—managed by kidneys
Upper lip right under the nose	Sexual organs
	excess caffeine can lead to heart irritations
Cheeks	Stomach
Lower cheeks	Lungs
Creases from nose to sides of mouth	Colon: ascending, transverse and descending
Mouth corners	Digestive system, stomach
Dry lips, cracked or sores	Flora: Probiotics are deficient
	Parasites, constipation
Upper Lip	Small Intestine
Lower Lip	Large Intestine
Chin (redness, acne, scars, growths)	Reproductive System
Wrinkles and dryness	Dehydration—poor absorption of water

FOODS TO KEEP YOUR SKIN BEAUTIFUL AND LENGTHEN YOUR LIFE

There are a number of supportive healthy diets to choose from these days such as the vegan diet, The Paleo diet, macrobiotic diet, raw food diet, The Ecology diet, the Ketogenic Diet and so on. They all provide basic sound nutrition that can lengthen your life, can help prevent age-related chronic health conditions and provide for healthy skin care.

For example, the basic foods in the Paleo diet are similar to foods that are generally regarded as a healthier alternative by avoiding the processed foods, sugar, grains and dairy. Foods that are considered to be okay to eat include: Vegetables, Fruits, Lean Meats, Seafood, Nuts & Seeds, and Healthy Fats. Foods to avoid are Dairy, Grains, Processed Food and Sugars, Legumes, Starches and Alcohol.

In the **Body Ecology Diet** Donna Gates strongly promotes a gluten-free, sugar-free, Probiotics-rich way to eat. She specifically designed a program to help cleanse and repair the inner ecosystem—the gut. She along with many others in the nutritional health field, have said disease begins in the gut. This same statement can just as well be applied to the skin—so I like to add: 'Skin conditions also begin in your gut.'

ANOTHER DIET—THE HIGH-FAT DIET MAY ALSO LENGTHEN YOUR LIFE

Dr. Mercola reports how numerous studies have shown that lowering your caloric intake may slow down your aging, help prevent age-related chronic diseases, and of course, extend your life. As you age, your levels of glucose, insulin and triglycerides tend to gradually creep upward. Basically the studies showed that those who lowered their insulin, by restricted calorie diets are living longer due to improved insulin regulation. Insulin resistance is a major factor in many chronic illnesses (lots of sugar and grains in one's diet) and is now being identified as a way that accelerates your aging. As a matter of fact, cancer cells thrive off of glucose but do NOT have the adaptability to survive off of Good fats. This is the basis of the Ketogenic diet.

Dr. Mercola writes: *"A 2010 study examined the effects of a high-fat diet on typical markers of aging. Study participants were given a high-fat, low-carbohydrate diet with adequate protein, and the results were health improvements across the board. Serum leptin decreased by an average of eight percent, insulin by 48 percent, fasting glucose by 40 percent, triglycerides by nearly eight percent, and free T3 (thyroid hormone) by almost six percent."*

> …our longevity depends more on what we are eating than on how much we are eating.

A Ketogenic diet is a diet that stresses a high consumption of healthy fats and low carbs. It requires that 50 to 70 percent of your food intake come from beneficial fats, such as coconuts and coconut oil, grass-pastured butter, olives and olive oil, organic pastured eggs, avocado, and raw nuts (raw pecans and almonds) and macadamia nuts which are particularly beneficial as they are low in protein and omega-6 fat.

From the amount of studies in nutrition alone, it is showing us that our longevity depends more on what we are eating than on how much we are eating. Perhaps a simple rule of thumb is to maintain a balanced, low caloric diet without any processed foods. Generally, include 40 percent complex carbohydrates, 20–30 percent lean protein and 40–50 percent good fat, depending upon your activity level and state of wellness.

> What you eat needs to be number one on your list for your health & beauty. Processed foods, sugary foods, and soft drinks,—all loaded with sugars and simple carbs—do not belong in any health regimen—especially in skin are, as they wrinkle the skin. Furthermore, they do not belong in a cancer-preventative diet. These foods turn into fuel for cancers.

Of course it is important to know your body's needs and to listen to your body, as it will give you the necessary feedback in regards to your food combinations. Know and understand your unique biochemistry and your genetics. This way you can adjust your food consumption accordingly.

Even with a healthy, organic diet, we may not get enough essential vitamins and minerals due to such conditions as depleted soil and imperfect growing conditions. You can supply your nutritional requirements by adding a variety of 'super-foods' to your daily intake. One simple way to increase raw, live super foods is in doing your own sprouting. Sprouting programs have literally 'sprouted' in the raw food community and there is a tremendous advantage for you to include this into your dietary regime. It's fairly easy to do and the nourishing sprouts can be added to your smoothies, salads or eat them as they are as a snack. They are a wholesome, hearty food that can provide you with a high amount of enzymes (See enzymes: why they are critical).

Vitamins provide potent combinations of antioxidants and healing agents that boost the skin's ability to make you look your glowing best. Here are some of the most important vitamins for skin care- where many of the foods are listed so that you can increase those foods as well.

ENZYMES: FIRST PLEASE!

Digestive enzymes are more important that we realize as the stomach is the center for all foods to be digested so that the nutrients can be assimilated. Unfortunately, starting at about the age of 30, the body's secretion of enzymes begins to gradually decline for a variety of reasons such as stress, poor food combinations, chemical toxins and medication. By the time a person reaches his/her senior years the enzyme decline is usually quite significant. This has a major adverse affect on the digestive process and assimilation of food.

The elderly are commonly known to have major digestive disturbances which lead to more deficiencies and further health decline.

Since 70% of the immune system lies in the gut, low enzyme production becomes a contributing factor to many age-related health conditions including osteoporosis, which is caused primarily by insufficient assimilation of proteins, calcium and other minerals. But it's not just the elderly who suffer from digestive complaints; younger individuals are suffering from insufficient digestive enzymes as well.

Buying antacids is not the solution for those who are in fact suffering with digestive complaints. Individuals are suffering instead from an enzyme deficiency (and from improper chewing of their food) than from excess stomach acid. Dull skin, hair loss, rashes, headaches, fatigue and weak nails are a few of the symptoms of low enzyme production. Dr. Oz presents an on-line simple low enzyme test that basically outlines the above mentioned symptoms. Anyone exhibiting these symptoms would be best to supplement their diets with food enzymes.

Digestive enzyme secretion starts first, in the mouth (part of the saliva), then second, by the stomach, and finally released into the small intestines from the liver and pancreas. Eating live foods (edible essential oils are live foods too) and raw, green foods will help to raise enzyme production as well as supplementation with food enzymes. For most of us, this is the first nutritional concern that is best to correct. Otherwise the vitamin, mineral absorption will be minimal and impaired.

VITAMINS—NURTURE YOUR SKIN

Excerpts from **Naturally Healthy Skin** by Stephanie Tourles

Vitamin A and Pro-Vitamin A (Beta-Carotene) are Fat-Soluble Antioxidants:
Some good sources are: liver (Especially fish liver oil), blue-green algae, pumpkin and winter squashes, alfalfa, carrots, cayenne pepper, dandelion greens, parsley, spinach, apricots, beet greens, broccoli, sweet potatoes, kale, lettuce, endive, cantaloupe, watermelon, tomatoes.

Skin benefits: Essential for growth and maintenance of epithelial (skin) tissue and proper functioning of mucous membranes. Vitamin A helps to prevent dry skin and premature aging. Speeds healing of acne and vision problems and boosts the immune system.

Deficiency symptoms: Can be the cause of early wrinkles, acne, pimples, blackheads, psoriasis and itching, scaly, cracked skin, loss of elasticity and enlarged pores.

Vitamin D Is a Fat-Soluble Antioxidant
Some good sources are: fish liver oils, salmon, tuna, alfalfa, watercress, egg yolks, and sunshine.

Skin benefits: Slows premature aging, and enhances bone mineralization and calcium absorption. Combined with vitamin A, it helps to remove acne.

Deficiency symptoms: Can be the cause of lack of vitality, slow growth and osteoporosis, weak teeth, bones, hair and nails.

Vitamin E is a Fat-Soluble Antioxidant

Some good sources are: cold-pressed vegetable oils, whole grains, eggs, alfalfa, parsley, sprouted seeds, nuts, fresh wheat germs, green leafy vegetables.

Skin benefits: Slows premature aging, protects eye and skin tissue, blocks formation of tumors, speeds skin healing, oxygenates tissues and promotes red blood cell formation.

Deficiency symptoms: Degeneration of epithelial cells in organs. This can cause collagen shrinkage, premature aging, easy bruising, lethargy, and more, rough and dry, tired skin and poor muscle tone.

B-Complex Vitamins are Water Soluble Nutrients

If you must supplement, be sure to take one that supplies the entire complex. Some good sources are: lean beef, chicken egg yolks, Brewer's Yeast, whole grains, alfalfa, almonds, sunflower seeds, green vegetables, fresh wheat germs, molasses, peas, beans.

Skin benefits: It is called the anti-stress vitamin! Helps prevent premature aging and acne. Promotes circulation and metabolism. Essential for wound healing. Aids new cell growth, increases vitality.

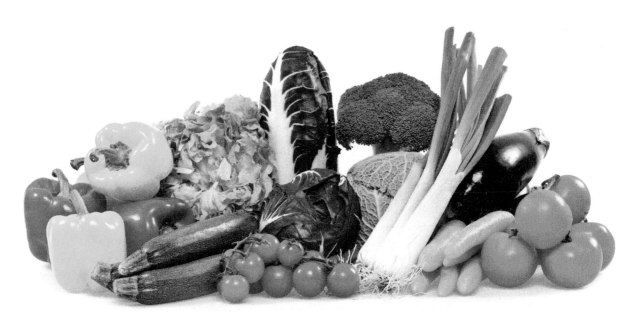

Deficiency symptoms: Sore mouth and lips; eczema; skin lesions; dandruff; pale complexion; pigmentation problems; premature wrinkles; premature aging; cracks around lips; oily, rashy skin and slow healing of skin.

Niacin (B-3) – is extremely beneficial for skin rejuvenation and the removal of toxins from fatty tissue. It helps to improve the skin's circulation.

Vitamin B-6 – is excellent for acne, anti-aging pollution, stress and beautiful skin.

Biotin (another B vitamin) – helps with hair loss, dermatitis, eczema, dandruff and seborrhea. Found in raspberries, grapefruit, tomatoes and nuts.

Vitamin C Is a Water Soluble Antioxidant
Some good sources are: citrus fruits, berries, pineapples, apples, persimmons, broccoli, green leafy vegetables, bell (especially red) and hot peppers, currants, papayas. Orange essential oil, Lime oil, Citrus Fresh essential oil (8 drops on abdomen)

Skin benefits: Helps produce collagen in connective tissue. Strengthens capillary walls, speeds healing, and helps battle environmental stress and toxins.

Deficiency symptoms: Easy bruising which does not go away, spongy gums, wrinkles, sagging skin, premature aging, slow healing, poor skin tone, cellulite.

Summary Vitamin Intake:
- **Vitamin A** – at least 5,000 IU daily. To construct new skin tissue, include at least 25,000 IU for three months, then to 15,000 IU daily.
- **Vitamin B** – complex (containing all B vitamins in a balanced tablet)
- **Vitamin C** – average of 3,000 to 5,000 mg daily throughout the day.
- **Vitamin E** – (mixed tocopherols preferred) 400 to 800 IU a day.

MINERALS

Apart from vitamins, essential minerals are important and considered even more important as they act as the catalyst for every function in the body. Minerals are the building blocks of beautiful skin! Four minerals in particular are necessary for the proper growth of healthy, luminous, resilient skin: iodine, silica, sulfur and zinc. Supplementing minerals in a liquid form

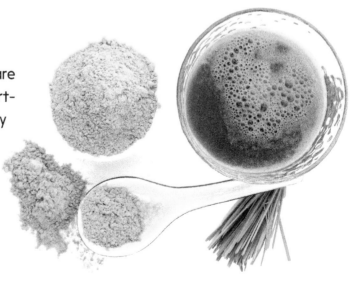

is ideal in maximizing absorption, such as found in Mineral Essence™ from Young Living or liquid minerals found in health food stores.

Multi Greens™

A proprietary blend of herbs and essential oils (a whole food mineral-rich nutrient) is an exclusive supplement available from Young Living.

It is a nutritious chlorophyll formula designed to boost vitality by working with the glandular, nervous, and circulatory systems. It contains ingredients that help cleanse the blood and support the immune, thyroid and digestive systems to relieve stress and promote energy metabolism and glucose utilization.

MultiGreens is made with Spirulina, alfalfa sprouts, barley grass, bee pollen, eleuthero, Pacific kelp and therapeutic-grade essential oils. According to the **_Essential Oils Desk Reference_** book published by Essential Science Publishing, each of these ingredients listed on the following page was better absorbed into the blood stream when the essential oils were added to the formula.

- **Spirulina** is a source of chlorophyll, a magnesium-rich pigment that has been linked to improved energy and metabolism. Spirulina has been used as a tonic, purifier and detoxifier. It targets the immune system, liver, kidneys, blood, intestinal flora and cardiovascular systems.
- **Barley grass** juice concentrate is a powerful antioxidant that is rich in minerals.
- **Bee pollen** is high in protein and low in fat and sodium. It is loaded with vitamins and minerals, including potassium, calcium, magnesium, zinc, manganese, copper and B vitamins.
- **Eleuthero root**, also known as Siberian Ginseng Root, enhances physical and mental vitality and endurance, reduces stress and strengthens lymphocyte formation.
- **L-arginine** is an amino acid that promotes circulation in the small capillaries of our tissues, allowing greater nutrient absorption and cellular metabolism.
- **L-cysteine** is an amino acid that supports healthy liver function and healthy hair.
- **L-tyrosine** is an amino acid necessary for the manufacture of thyroid hormones and can be taken alone or as a component of a nutritional supplement which is the best way for it to be taken. It also supports the production of neuro-transmitters, such as dopamine and serotonin.
- **Choline bitartrate** has been used in the treatment of Alzheimer's disease and many liver disorders, including elevated cholesterol levels, viral hepatitis, and cirrhosis. It is essential for liver health.

- Pacific Kelp contains iodine that helps prevent goiters, thyroid hormonal imbalance and estrogen imbalance.

Unique addition to **Young Living's MultiGreens** is the following essential oils:

- **Melissa** (Melissa Officinalis) is anti-inflammatory and energizing.
- **Lemon** (Citrus limon) helps dissolve cholesterol and increase lymphatic (immune) function.
- **Lemongrass** (Cymbopogon flexuous) is antiparasitic, antifungal, antibacterial promotes digestion and clears bladder infections
- **Rosemary CT cineol** (Rosmarinus Officinalis) helps prevent Candida and balance the endocrine system.

Alkalime® – A proprietary blend of essential oils & mineral powder

Another important and specially designed mineral powder that contains high-alkaline salts is called **AlkaLime**®, a Young Living product. It is a precisely-balanced alkaline mineral complex formulated to neutralize acidity in the digestive system, blood and the body and maintain desirable pH levels in the body, a cornerstone of health. Infused with lemon and lime essential oils and organic whole lemon powder, **AlkaLime**® also features enhanced effervescence and **biochemic tissue cell salts** for increased effectiveness. A balanced pH helps to reduce yeast and fungus in the body. **AlkaLime** helps with a host of symptoms related to acid-based yeast fungus dominance: headaches, overweight, low resistance, allergies, mood swings, indigestion, ulcers, Candida and so on. **AlkaLime** combines tissue cell salts in a unique pleasant tasting way.

These include:

- **Sodium** (as bicarbonate, phosphate and sulfate);
- **Calcium** (as carbonate, phosphate and sulfate);
- **Magnesium phosphate**; and
- **Potassium** (as bicarbonate, chloride, phosphate and sulfate).

Also contains these essential oils:

- **Lemon Essential Oil** (Citrus limon) consists of 68 percent d-limonene, a powerful antioxidant; and may be beneficial for the skin, is antiseptic, promotes leukocyte formation, improves memory and increases immune function. It has cleansing and purifying properties.

- **Lime Essential Oil** (Citrus auantiifolia) decongests the lymphatic system, is a natural immune system booster; and supports natural weight loss when used in conjunction with a weight management program and/or exercise program. May aid in mental clarity, reduces stress and may also support healthy skin when applied to the skin.

Biochemic Cell Salts

Dr. Schussler discovered the health-supporting effect of several mineral cell salts that were developed homeopathically for the assimilation by the cells of the body. He identified the 12 different cell salts present in every cell in the human body. He maintained that if these specialist cells become deficient in one or more of these salts certain symptoms and disease will result. **When the correct salts are replenished in the body, health will be restored.**

Three of the salts that pertain to skin care in **AlkaLime** have been highlighted below:

Calcium sulphate is found in bile; promotes continual blood cleansing. When deficient in the body, toxic build-up occurs in the form of **skin disorders**, respiratory clog, boils and ulcerations and slow healing. Present in connective tissue and in liver cells. Used for cellular regeneration; infection due to pus; pimples, sore throats, colds, pancreatic, liver and kidney disturbances; frontal headaches with nausea; excessive sensitivity of nerves as well as cravings for fruit and acids.

Kali Sulph or Potassium sulphate is an **oxygen-carrier** for the skin. A deficiency of this cell salt causes a deposit on the tongue and slimy nasal, eye, ear and mouth secretions. Found in epidermis and epithelial cells. Potassium sulphate carries oxygen to the cells. Used for hot flashes; chills; weariness; heaviness; giddiness; boxed in feelings; stomach catarrh; inflammatory conditions; eruptions of the skin; shifting pains; palpitations; anxiety; fear; sadness; toothaches; headaches and pains in limbs that tend to increase indoors especially in warm and close rooms or in the warm summer air; yellow/slimy catarrhal discharges; dandruff; psoriasis and diseases of the nails (rough or ribbed).

Calcium phosphate is an important constituent of the bones, skeletal system, especially the teeth, the knees and the joints, the gall bladder *and the skin*. The body requires larger amounts of Calc phos. than any other, especially during childhood and growth spurts, or when recovering from broken bones. Skeletal problems such as rickets, curvature of the spine and tooth decay respond well to this cell salt. Elderly people are particularly responsive to Calc phos. because it not only adds calcium to the system but improves gastric digestive function so all vitamins and minerals are better assimilated. This cell salt has an affinity for the bones, teeth, glands, nerves, blood, gastric juices, and connective tissues. It is an excellent restorative remedy for the convalescent.

AlkaLime is best to be taken 1 hour before meals, mixed in water. Drink immediately.

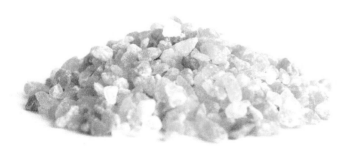

Iodine

Good sources are: fish, shellfish, sunflower seeds, kelp, seaweed, iodized salt, sea salt.

Skin benefits: Aides in healing skin infections, increases oxygen consumption and metabolic rate in the skin. Helps prevent roughness and premature wrinkling.

Deficiency symptoms: Slowed growth and healing, slowed metabolism, poor skin tone, dry and wrinkled skin

Contraindication: Iodine may aggravate acne skin.

Best found in MultiGreens, Mineral Essence from Young Living, also high quality iodine drops are available either from leading health stores or on-line such as what can be found on www.Drbrownstein.com/Overcoming-Thyroid-Disorders-p/overcomingt.htm.

Silica

Good sources are: horsetail, nettle, Echinacea root, dandelion root, alfalfa, kelp, flaxseed, oat straw, barley grass, wheat grass, apples, berries, burdock root, beets, onion, almonds, peanuts, sunflower seed and grapes.

Skin benefits: Aids in collagen formation, strengthens bones and skin tissues, helps prevent wrinkles, brittle nails, and hair.

Deficiency symptoms: Premature wrinkles, lack of skin tone, sagging skin, flabbiness, dull hair.

Contained in Mineral Essence from Young Living and often found in liquid minerals at health food stores.

Sulfur (MSM)

Sulfur or MSM (methyl sulfonyl methane) is considered by many nutritionists as the **foundational beauty** mineral and the best cosmetic in the world. One of the best sources of nutritional sulfur is methylsulfonylmethane (MSM). Our body needs it for many critical functions and doesn't get enough of it through our food—it's considered just as important as water. Cooking destroys this mineral and plants lose it quickly soon after they are picked. MSM aids in the proper formation of proteins associated with connective tissues, hormones and antibodies plus the formation of collagen.

Collagen is important for skin integrity and elasticity. It is critical to proper skin health, hair, nail growth and liver functions. Helps to boost immunity, natural detoxification, helps to alleviate pollen and food allergies, reduces lactic acid buildup and possibly reduces muscle, leg and back cramps. Sulfur also regulates the sodium/potassium electrolyte balance in and out of the cells. Helps to relieve constipation and helps to heal burns and scars.

Some of the best sources are Pine bark, pine needles, pine nuts, aloe vera, turnips, dandelion greens, radishes, horseradish, string beans, onion, garlic, arugula, cabbage, celery, kale, watercress, soybeans, fresh fish, lean meats, eggs, asparagus.

Skin benefits: Sulphur has been called the best beauty mineral. Helps repair damaged skin by stimulating production of collagen, helps for scar tissue and helps with wrinkle repair.

It is well researched by Dr. Ronald Lawrence for arthritic pain, joint and muscle pain, reducing inflammation and by breaking up scar tissue. It increases blood circulation as well as maintaining acid-alkaline balance. Keeps skin clear and smooth.

Deficiency symptoms: Dry scalp, rashes, eczema, acne, scaly skin, weak nails, allergies, poor digestion, joint pain or inflammation.

Best found in **Mineral Essence**, or **Sulferzyme™** (a proprietary blend by Young Living) which contains MSM and Chinese Wolfberry. It is best to be taken 15–30 minutes before a meal. MSM can also be found in health food stores but quality MSM is an issue—so, knowing the reputation of the company becomes critical.

Zinc
50mg. 1–2x a day

Good sources are: barley grass, alfalfa, yellow dock root, Echinacea root, kelp, dulce, fresh wheat germ, pumpkin seeds, sunflower seeds, Brewer's Yeast, milk, eggs, fish, oysters, green leafy vegetables, onions, beans, nuts, macadamia nuts, esp. flaxseed oil and walnuts.

Skin benefits: Aids in wound healing, promotes cell growth, boosts immunity, helps treat acne when it is combined with vitamins A and B. Zinc can help fight acne because it's involved in metabolizing testosterone, which affects the production of an oily substance caused sebum, a primary cause of acne. Zinc also assists in new-cell production and the sloughing off of dead skin, which gives the skin a nice glow.

Zinc can help repair DNA damage and prevents wrinkling, stretch marks etc. It is essential for skin and collagen.

Deficiency symptoms: Slow healing, dandruff, lowered resistance to infections, loss of skin elasticity, wrinkles, stretch marks, white spots on nails, hair loss (Also found in Mineral Essence).

Add Mineral Essence to also obtain your trace minerals. Mineral Essence contains purified water, honey, royal jelly, trace minerals, essential oils of lemon, cinnamon bark and peppermint.

OTHER KEY MINERALS:

Selenium

Selenium is an essential trace element that works with Vitamin E, to produce a potent antioxidant, called glutathione (See section on glutathione). This mineral helps to promote a healthy immune system that helps us fight off illness and is important for healthy skin. It also helps the regulation of thyroid hormones.

Experts say selenium plays a key role in the health of skin cells. Some studies show that even skin damaged by the sun may suffer fewer consequences if selenium levels are high. Researchers at Edinburgh University showed that when levels of selenium were high, skin cells were less likely to suffer the kind of oxidative damage that can increase the risk of cancer. The results were published in 2003 in both the **British Journal of Dermatology** and the journal **Clinical and Experimental Dermatology**.

Another group of French researchers found that oral doses of selenium, along with copper, vitamin E and vitamin A could prevent sunburn cell formation in human skin. Good Sources are: found in eggs, organic whole grains, beans, onions, tomatoes, **Brazil nuts**, mushrooms, garlic.

Deficiency symptoms: premature aging, loss of skin elasticity, dandruff.

Dr. Oz states that eating selenium rich foods such as mushrooms and Brazil nuts with iodized salt can help recharge a sluggish thyroid, promoting increased energy and weight loss. He also suggests that eating cod is beneficial to the skin. Cod contains selenium and thus can help safeguard our skin from sun damage and cancer.

Calcium
1,000 mg./1200 mg. over the age of 50

It is vital to the health of your bones, teeth and bodily organs, including the skin.

Skin benefits: Calcium plays a role in regulating the skin's many functions. Most calcium in the skin is found in the epidermis, or the outermost layer of skin. Calcium in the epidermis helps the body regulate how fast it generates new skin cells to replace old ones and how quickly it sheds old skin cells.

Deficiency symptoms: weak hair, teeth, nails, PMS, insomnia.

Skin that does not have enough calcium stored in the epidermis may appear fragile, thin and dry. Deficiency can manifest itself in dryness, itching, premature wrinkling and an increased tendency to develop skin cancers.

Calcium is important in regulating the production of an antioxidant called catalase. Catalase, along with other important antioxidants prevents the DNA damage that damages the texture of skin, and minimizes damage to collagen and elastin.

Magnesium
400 mg.

Skin benefits: It is the **fourth most abundant mineral** in our bodies Magnesium is directly responsible for over 300 biochemical reactions, it is an essential electrolyte mineral required for all life.

- Magnesium slows down the aging process in the skin because magnesium stabilizes DNA and RNA which are both negatively charged and are attracted to the positively charged magnesium.
- Magnesium is also needed to **remineralize teeth**—Magnesium deficiency causes an unhealthy balance of phosphorous and calcium in saliva, which damages teeth. Alkalizes the body—Magnesium helps return the body's pH balance.
- Hydrates—Magnesium is a necessary electrolyte essential for proper hydration.
- Helps to relieve constipation—Magnesium can be used to cleanse the bowels of toxins.
- Enzyme function—Enzymes: helps in Hair re-growth
- Anti allergic: Magnesium has the capacity to detoxify the epidermis and cleanse the skin to relieve those areas of the skin that are prone to allergic reactions.
- Anti wrinkle: Magnesium is very effective in reducing **fine lines around your eyes and wrinkles on forehead.**
- Pimples: magnesium helps combat break outs or acne on your skin.
- Magnesium can avert heart disease and many more health benefits.

David Wolfe author, educator, nutritionist, says in his book ***Eating for Beauty***, that *"The beauty of our hair, skin and nails depends on how mineralized we are."* That means eating more dark green, leafy vegetables that are high in chlorophyll. So you can now look forward to a yummy green spinach smoothie for breakfasts and more green leafy veggies throughout the day.

Spinach provides us with a powerful source of magnesium. Seaweed, pumpkin and sunflower seeds are also good healthy sources of magnesium. However, there is a significant magnesium loss whenever we cook or boil these foods. So include many raw foods in your diet as much as possible, which is easier to do when combining them into a smoothie or juicing them. **Mag**nify your beauty with **mag**nesium enriched foods in your diet every day!

Deficiency symptoms: stress-related skin problems, low vitality, low muscle tone, low calcium and vitamin C metabolism, tense muscles, irritability.

Potassium

Good Sources are: bananas, sea vegetables, dried fruits, almonds, watercress and green peppers.

Skin benefits: Potassium is the **third most abundant mineral** in the human body and a powerful element in improving health.

Apart from acting as an electrolyte, this mineral is required for preventing hair loss, relief from cramps, keeping the heart, brain, kidney, muscle tissue and other important organ systems of the human body in good condition.

Potassium keeps the skin moisturized and hydrated internally. So, to cure dry skin, start eating potassium rich fruits and vegetables like bananas, potatoes, etc.

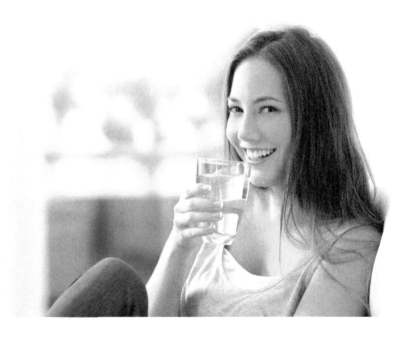

Potassium also supports the growth of new skin cells. If your skin does not produce enough new cells, it will appear cracked and dull. Also, blemishes and scars fade away after some time if the natural growth of skin cells is balanced. It acts as a ph level balancer for the skin. It absorbs water molecules from the environment and hydrates the skin. Potassium hydroxide is used in a lot of cosmetics and skin care products for this reason.

Deficiency symptoms: muscular weakness, poor digestion, anxiety, stressed, dry skin, acne, dermatitis.

Potassium-deficient people may also experience high blood pressure, pain in their intestines, swelling in their glands and diabetes as serious side effects of this deficiency.

WATER

It's not a surprise that water is a very important nutrient for so many functions. When your water intake does not equal your output, you can become dehydrated. Fluid losses are accentuated in warmer climates, during strenuous exercise, in high altitudes, and in older adults, whose sense of thirst may not be as sharp.

Your body is composed of about 70% water. Besides its many functions of these bodily fluids that include digestion, absorption, circulation, creation of saliva, transportation of nutrients, and maintenance of body temperature, the skin requires water to maintain hydration. If your skin is not getting the sufficient amount of water, the lack of hydration will present itself by turning your skin dry, tight and flaky. Dry skin has less resilience and is more prone to wrinkling.

Fluoride's Dangers

But there is a danger! It is called Fluoride. Fluoride, as other chemical toxins, is a poison and is often found in drinking water as it is added to purify city water.

Fluoride is a corrosive acid called Hydrofluorosilicic Acid – captured in the air pollution control devices of the phosphate fertilizer industry. It is a toxic waste by-product of phosphate fertilizer production.

The EPA has classified these 3 forms of fluoride as toxins: fluorosilicate acid, sodium silico-fluoride, and sodium fluoride (that is used in dentistry) – BUT all are waste products of the nuclear, aluminum, and now mostly the phosphate (fertilizer) industries. Sodium Fluoride is a pesticide! EPA lists fluoride as a contaminant and is also an **"endocrine disruptor."**

Other harmful side effects:

- Causes thyroid damage
- Calcifies the pineal
- Causes weight gain
- Edema
- Kidney disease, kidney failure
- Hair loss
- Depression

- Aggression, aches, pains, skin problems, bone deformities (likely including "arthritis" and spontaneous fractures)
- Sexual/erectile dysfunction, memory loss, weakness, fatigue
- Heart disease, irritability, cancer, digestive disorders

Dr. Jennifer Luke's study on *Fluoride Deposition in the Aged Human Pineal Gland* has shown for the first time that fluoride readily accumulates in the aged human pineal gland. This is critical in how the pineal gland is hampered by calcification and is the cause of many diseases including Alzheimer's (More on the Pineal gland below).

How much clean, purified or natural spring water to drink?

On average, drinking at least 6–8 glasses a day will help rid the body and skin of toxins and keep the skin hydrated.

MORE ON ANTIOXIDANTS

Many researchers point out the importance of using antioxidants to stop free radicals in their tracks. This is a full-time job to keep cells healthy, your skin gorgeous and your body disease free.

Just imagine slicing an apple and leaving it on your kitchen counter uncovered. Over a short period of time, it begins to oxidize and turn brown. This same cell deterioration happens inside your body, known as free radical damage. Free radicals, an unstable oxygen molecule, that punches holes in cell membranes damaging cellular DNA, pave the way for cancer and diseases of aging. Only antioxidants (like vitamins A, C and E) can neutralize free radicals.

Dr. Perricone highly stresses the consumption of the freshest fruits and vegetables several times a day. Since this may be challenging to do at times, a vitamin/mineral program is recommended.

ANTIOXIDANT GLUTATHIONE:

Glutathione is the body's most important defense against free radicals. It defends the cells against chemical toxins, heavy metals, radiation, pollution, disease, **aging and oxidative stress**. Declining levels of glutathione in the body increases vulnerability to over 70 major diseases. **Glutathione** is a naturally occurring substance that is an anti-oxidant, detoxifier and immune system booster.

Oxidative stress is the damage caused to our cells as the result of normal oxidative processes occurring all the time in our bodies.

Citrus oils enhance *Glutathione* production in the body, as does **thyme oil**, Ningxia red berries and juice and many of the immune stimulating oils. Glutathione patches have been created by a company to deliver on-going support of this critical nutrient.

Other nutrients that have been researched for anti-aging purposes include:
L-carnosine: Maca root, sea buckthorn oil as a supplement, vitamin B-3 (great for eye shadows and puffiness), chromium, Ningxia berries, chlorella.

OTHER ANTIOXIDANTS

- **Co Q10** – 30 to 100 mg.
  - Coenzyme Q10 is a powerful antioxidant most concentrated in the heart muscle, which requires the most fuel. May help prevent or treat heart weakness. It also helps to reduce wrinkles. It helps neutralize harmful free radicals, which is one of the causes of aging.
  - Co Q10 is most depleted in the skin due to sun exposure. Thus, CoQ10 may boost skin repair and regeneration, protect the cell membrane and reduce free radical damage. Furthermore, CoQ10 can reduce UV cell damage.
  - Co Q10 is found in a number of products today—and is now available in a product called **MindWise™** by Young Living.

- **Alpha Lipoic Acid** – 100 mg.
  - Best for free radical damage, helps to prevent the glycosylation (sugar damage)
  - Clinical studies suggest ALA may help prevent nerve damage caused by free radicals often found in diabetes. ALA neutralizes free radicals in both the fatty and watery parts of cells, having the ability to zip in and out of cells, even those in the brain.
  - Can be found in most health food stores as a nutrient supplement.

- **Omega 3/6 oils** (2:1 ratio)
  The Omega-3s amazing benefits:
  - They're anti-inflammatory and anti-clotting
  - They prevent age-related cognitive decline
  - They lower triglycerides
  - They lower blood pressure
  - They slow age-related macular degeneration
  - They keep blood vessels flexible
  - They lower depression
  - They decrease joint stiffness in rheumatoid and osteo-arthritis
  - They're necessary for fetal and infant brain development

**New research now shows the benefits of
Omega 3 on lengthening the Telomeres.**

Essential fatty acids are important in preventing premature aging of the skin and for hormonal balance. Include borage seed oil, black currant oil and evening primrose oil or flaxseed oil in your supplementation. Salmon is a good food source.

Omega Gize 3 – is a brand from Young Living that contains Omega 3

You can get all your Omega-3 from green leafy vegetables, legumes, flax seeds, Chia seeds (they have now been discovered to have the highest level of Omega 3—higher than flax seeds), or walnuts, highly purified fish oil supplements, or algae-sourced Omega 3 supplements.

"The main result of our study is that patients with high levels of Omega-3 fish oil in the blood appear to have a slowing of the biological aging process over five years as measured by the change in telomere length. It's also the first study that shows that a dietary factor may be able to slow down telomere shortening."
RAMIN FARZANEH-FAR, M.D

Hyaluronic acid – Another anti-aging supplement addition in skin care:

Hyaluronic acid is the latest rave in a nutrient supplement for the skin. Hyaluronic acid is a gel that is found in the soft tissue throughout your body. It keeps your cells healthy, moisturized and resilient. Hyaluronic acid supports the formation and maintenance of collagen (the principal protein in human skin, bone, cartilage, joints, tendons and connective tissue).

Our bodies produce less hyaluronic acid as we age. By age 40, diminished supplies of hyaluronic acid leaves us with aches, pains and wrinkles. Lane Labs conducted a small study using hyaluronic acid combination focusing particularly on wrinkles, puffiness and sagging around the eyes. There was a significant reduction of wrinkles and other signs of aging after just two weeks of supplementation. It works deep down – considered to be an inside face-lift. Sold by two companies, Synovo Derma from Allergy Research Groups and Toki from Lane Labs

Astragalus – In a study entitled: "Effects of Astragalus root on the expression of P16 mRNA and telomere of human dermal fibroblasts by serum pharmacology" researchers found that: Astragalus root serum can postpone senescence by increasing the activity of SOD, depressing the expression of P16 and inhibiting the shortening of telomeres. In other words, and simply said:

Astragalus root has a profound effect on the aging factor.

CLEANSING

"The only way to beauty is to clean out the garbage."
MARKUS ROTHKRANZ

Large Intestine – Cleanse your Colon first
First Place to Start in Cleansing!

Want beautiful skin — then you can't have a toxic bowel. The colon or the large intestine is the most important system for total health care and hence why it is linked to almost every disease we could have. For most people the colon or large intestine is their weakest link, as the saying goes: a chain is only as strong as its weakest link. As mentioned earlier in this chapter, disease begins in the gut and so do skin conditions.

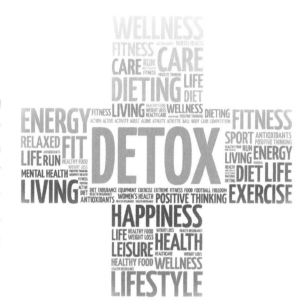

The large intestine system takes about 16 hours to finish the digestion of your food. It is not just for the removal of the `garbage` afterwards but plays a vital role in removing water and any remaining absorbable nutrients from the food before sending the indigestible matter to the rectum. It has the important job of extracting the nutrients and absorbing them into the bloodstream via the liver.

The colon absorbs vitamins that are created by the colonic bacteria, our friendly bacteria- utilizing vitamin K which is especially important as the daily ingestion of vitamin K is not normally enough to maintain adequate blood coagulation, vitamin B12, thiamine and riboflavin. So, if unhealthy processed food is eaten, not only is it of poor nutritional value, but it is acidic to the body. As a way to protect the intestinal lining, the body coats the food with mucus. This mucus coats our intestines eventually forming a hard mucoid plaque, which makes it very difficult for nutrients to be absorbed into our body. This is the perfect medium for parasites, fungus and bacteria to begin feasting on the feces. The colon stores fecal matter in the rectum until it can be discharged via the anus in defecation. Toxic bowel content means that toxic substances are re-absorbed into our bloodstream—poisoning the liver, kidneys and other bodily systems including the skin. This is called auto-intoxication, a way of slow self-poisoning, coined by Dr. Bernard Jensen, a well-recognized herbalist, iridologist who specialized in bowel cleansing.

Bowel cleansing will help with so many ailments, such as breathing, heart conditions, depression, wrinkles, cancer, anger, hormones, skin issues, fertility, liver, energy issues to name a few. The way to correct this situation is to cleanse our colons.

The colon is also very vulnerable to stress, tension and emotions. In the Oriental system of health, the bowel or colon is all about letting go and, it is also the repository for grief, sadness, shock and holding on to past emotions. Cleansing the colon will also help to release toxic emotional baggage. On a physical level, Vitamin K1 is essential for healthy bowel function. Vitamin K is found chiefly in leafy green vegetables such as dandelion greens (which contain 778.4 µg per 100 g, or 741% of the recommended daily amount), kale (531 micrograms per half cup) , spinach, (444 micrograms per half cup) collards, swiss chard, lettuce etc. The absorption is greater when accompanied by fats such as butter, coconut oil or other healthy oils. Some fruits such as avocado, kiwifruit and grapes, are also high in vitamin K. Eat or drink your GREENS is certainly not just a fad but a necessary health habit.

A healthy colon needs to be pH balanced (approx. 6.4 pH), (hence our greens) in order for healthy bacteria (called Probiotics) to flourish and keep the unfriendly microbes in check.

Some helpful tips for Bowel Cleansing:
1. **Increase your Greens** – make Green Smoothies every day as part of your life. Add dark green leafy vegetables to your smoothie.

2. **Increase your fiber** – such as apples (organic only); so perhaps the cliché of "an apple a day keeps the doctor away", can be elaborated to: keeps the bugs away.

3. **Do a full bowel cleanse** at least 4 times a year using a Colon Cleanse high fiber herbal and essential oil combination.

4. **Add other juices to cleanse:** celery, cucumber, carrot, spinach, kale, lemon juice, lime juice

5. **Increase digestive enzymes,** Magnesium` and Probiotics into your regimen every day.

6. **Add Celery Seed essential oil** – Antioxidant, diuretic, antibacterial, liver protectant. It is helpful in digestion, liver cleansing and the urinary system. Helps to reduce cellulite deposits and researched for its ability to reduce blood pressure and cholesterol. Has a hormonal property, as it stimulates mother's milk.

   Add 2 drops to your smoothies or juices. Add 1 drop to your tea to help urinary function.

Negative emotions such as **frustration, anger and hostility** produce emotional toxins. The liver has difficulty in processing these emotional toxins, which are stored in the muscles and tissues of the body resulting in distress and disease.

7. **Chia Seeds** – increase these in your diet as they are a better source of Omega 3 and are very hydrating in the colon and acts as a great colon cleanser. Add to liquids, drink immediately before it gels.

8. **Add other cleansing essential oils** like: DiGize™ blend for digestive and bowel cleansing, Geranium, Release™ blend over abdomen to assist with emotional letting go as well.

LIVER AND YOUR SKIN

Having healthy, vibrant and beautiful skin also means having a healthy liver. The skin is a reflection of your liver and is often referred to as an outer liver. The word liver comes from the old English word for "life." To the Chinese, the liver is considered "the father of all organs."

The liver is the body's second largest organ; only the skin is larger and heavier. The liver performs many essential functions related to digestion, metabolism, immunity, and the storage of nutrients within the body.

One of the main functions of the liver is to maintain the level of fats in the bloodstream. For an average person, approximately 80% of the cholesterol is generated by the liver.

The liver is one of the most important detoxifying organs in the body. It is the most complicated organ with the greatest number of functions (known to have 5,000 chemical functions a day) transforming digested food into usable materials and disposing of waste substances; thus affecting every cell of our body. Over a liter of blood passes through the liver every minute. When the liver is overloaded, the skin excretes the toxins and poisons present in the body.

WHAT OVERLOADS THE LIVER?

- the pollutants in our food, air and water
- chemical food additives
- pharmaceutical drugs
- chlorination and fluoridation of water

- car exhaust
- pesticides; herbicides
- parasites, Candida, viruses, mold
- mercury amalgams
- denatured, processed foods
- tobacco smoke
- sugars
- and the worst of all, toxic emotions

Negative emotions such as **frustration, anger and hostility** produce emotional toxins. The liver has difficulty in processing these emotional toxins, which are stored in the muscles and tissues of the body resulting in distress and disease.

Out of the many functions that the liver performs, the most important is to produce bile, which helps in digestion through the process of emulsification of lipids. A sluggish liver produces less bile, causing many digestion problems.

Some of the symptoms of toxic or stressed liver include the following:

DIGESTIVE PROBLEMS		
skin irritations	heart burn	Constipation
blemishes	bloating	Loss of appetite
acne	general fatigue	Swollen feet or abdomen
rashes	loss of appetite	Bad breath
psoriasis	itching skin or hives	Heartburn
eczema	allergies	Body odor
brownish spots on the skin	depression and irritability	Intolerance to alcohol
nausea and abdominal swelling	yellow discoloration of the skin or eyes	dark-colored urine and loss of energy
Inability to digest fatty foods	Allergy to chemicals in paints, petrol, bleaches, etc.	

The liver is responsible for filtering out mutated hormones. A person with a sluggish liver would be quite affected by the hormonal imbalance and would exhibit symptoms such as:

- Sleep and mental disturbance
- Mental confusion
- Depression
- Sensitivity to medicines

For women, hormonal imbalance due to a sluggish liver causes:

- Heavy or clotted menstruation
- Irregular periods
- Fibroids in breast or uterus
- Hot flashes
- Cysts on ovaries
- Mood swings or any menopausal problems

The list of symptoms is exhaustive and varied—and I wanted to feature just enough of them to show you how important it is to keep your liver healthy and happy in order to obtain longevity, vitality and beautiful skin.

WAYS TO LOVE YOUR LIVER

Do's and Dont's

1. Avoid pharmaceutical medications as much as possible—too many chemicals harm your liver.

2. Street drugs cause serious damage and scar your liver permanently.

3. Avoid drowning your liver in alcohol.

4. Be especially cautious in mixing alcohol with drugs and medications. Best to avoid alcohol altogether.

5. Avoid using aerosol cleaners; your liver has to detoxify what you breathe in.

6. Bug sprays, paint sprays and all chemical sprays can harm your liver.

7. Be careful what gets onto your skin! Serious chemicals like insecticides and herbicides go through your skin to your liver, destroying some cells.

8. Avoid household cleaners in your laundry, dishes, furniture for many of the reasons listed above (see **Vibrational Cleaning** book for more details as to the harm these chemicals cause).

EAT FOR A HEALTHY LIVER—IT IS YOUR CHOICE!

Everything you eat must pass through your liver. You have only the liver that can purify your blood stream. So pay attention to your nutrition to keep a healthy liver which will give you a healthy you with youthful, radiant skin.

Choose to eat a well balanced diet (see youth foods).

Avoid deep fried and fatty foods, smoked, cured and salted foods.

Use high antioxidant essential oils, such as thyme oil, to raise glutathione levels in the liver (Haroun, et al., 2002).

Use alternative seasonings in your cooking such as lemon juice, onion, garlic, mustard, cloves, sage, oregano or thyme.

Increase your fiber (fresh fruits, vegetables: keep whole grains to a minimum or none at all). Eat moderate amounts of fruit instead of rich desserts and drinks. Avoid sugary foods. Excess sugar including fructose (sucrose is 50% fructose and recent research shows fructose causes the same major harmful effects), promotes free radical damage, cross-links with protein to form advanced glycation end-products or AGEs. These damaged proteins, impair cellular function and accelerate aging (Whitaker, May 2003).

Use fresh lemons and pure warm water upon arising in the morning. Lemon stimulates blood circulation, reduces arterial pressures, activates bile and intestinal secretions and produces a general feeling of well-being. Add a drop of lemon oil to the mixture.

DETOX FOR YOUR GALL-BLADDER (PULLS TOXINS)

Formula 1 by Markus Rothkranz

- Drink every day for several weeks
- Blend- orange, lemon, lime and grapefruit juice
- 3–5 cloves of garlic
- thumb sized piece of Ginger
- half cup of olive or hemp oil
- pinch of Celtic sea salt

This drink helps to purge the toxins, such as bacteria, parasites etc. and the ginger helps to keep the toxins flowing.

FORMULA 2

- Ingest every morning
- Add to a capsule: 5 drops each of Lemon, Tangerine and Grapefruit oil with 2–3 drops of Ledum oil – Repeat 2–3 x day before meals for 2–3 weeks

FORMULA 3

- Ingest Juva Cleanse oil (Special Young Living dietary blend) by adding 8–10 drops to a gel cap
- Can take 1–2 caps per day, for 2 weeks
- Also apply 6–10 drops of any of these oils:
- Juva Flex, Lemon, Ledum, hyssop, juniper, or Citrus Fresh oils over the gallbladder area 2–3 times daily
- Apply a warm compress and relax for 15 minutes

FORMULA 4

Apply topically, Juva Flex, 'special Young Living blend. JuvaFlex consists of the following oils:

- **Geranium** (Pelargonium graveolens) – improves bile flow from the liver, antispasmodic, improves liver, pancreas and kidney function.

- **Rosemary** (Rosmarinus officinalis) – beneficial as a toner for all skin conditions; decongests the liver. liver protecting, balances the endocrine system

- **Roman Chamomile** (Chamaemelum nobile) – expels toxins from the liver, strengthens the liver and beneficial for the skin.

- **Fennel** (Foeniculum vulgare) – stimulating to the circulatory system, increases bile, and hepatocyte function

- **Helichrysum** (Helichrysum italicum) – researched for regenerating tissue and nerves, helps to regulate cholesterol, stimulates liver cell function, and helps to clean plaque and debris from the veins and arteries.

- **Blue Tansy** (Tanacetum annuum) – cleanses the liver and calms the lymphatic system, also helps one to overcome anger and negative emotions.

JuvaFlex can be applied over the liver, along the back or on the reflex point on the feet.

Juva Cleanse consists of the following oils:

- **Ledum** (Ledum groenlandicum) – helps to digest fat cells in the liver and functions as an enzyme (chemical poisons are stored in the fat cells in the liver). Can be used for all types of skin problems.

- **Helichrysum** (Helichrysum italicum) – powerful chelating agent of metallics and chemicals. Studied for its ability to regenerate tissue and nerves, and improve circulation and skin conditions. Works synergistically with Ledum.

- **Celery Seed** (Apium graveolens) – used for bladder and kidney complaints, digestive ailments, acts as a natural diuretic of the liver to expedite the transport of wastes, also has a liver regenerating effect.

Juva Cleanse may be added to juice, water or capsule as a dietary supplement.

GLF (another special Young Living oil blend) stands for Gallbladder and Liver Flush consists of:

- **Grapefruit** decongesting and fat-dissolving, has anti-coagulant properties helps to improve the flow of bile to and from the liver.

- **Helichrysum** – stimulates liver cell function and removes plaque from veins and arteries (see above for more benefits)

- **Celery seed** – a powerful liver cleanser

- **Ledum** – helps to digest fat cells in the liver and functions as an enzyme (chemical poisons are stored in the fat cells in the liver). Improves bile function. Can be used for all types of skin problems.

- **Hyssop** – is a decongestant that is also anti-inflammatory, antiparasitic, anti-infectious

- **Spearmint** – has antispasmodic, anti-infectious, antiparasitic, antiseptic and anti-inflammatory properties. It has also been used to increase metabolism for fat burning. Can be applied in a gel cap as described in Formula 4.

SUPPLEMENTS

Other herbs that aid the liver that are very helpful for skin conditions are: herbal burdock, beet powder and juice, capsicum, cascara sagrada, dandelion, red clover, yellow dock, milk thistle and Oregon grape root.

Use as a tea or take as capsules. The following supplements are also very helpful: vitamins A, B-Complex, D, E, black currant oil, evening primrose oil, chlorophyll and alpha-lipoic acid.

ANOTHER ANTI-AGING DISCOVERY—STEM CELLS

One of the biggest breakthroughs taking place in anti-aging has to do with stem cells. Many researchers are claiming that we're beginning to see the end of most diseases because stem cells offer treatments, and even cures. Stem cell research and treatments are gaining tremendous momentum in all areas of medicine.

The developments in anti-aging stem cell facial serums are now making headlines in the search for `that Fountain of Youth.' The same molecules that are found in plants that don't age are now being identified and used to activate the skin's stem cells. The understanding is simply this: that applying these anti-aging molecules on your skin, gives the message to the skin cells to reproduce younger, fresher cells.

Are there essential oils that can stimulate stem cells?

Yes, indeed essential oils do have the capacity in stimulating stem cells. So far, extensive research on Frankincense essential oil has shown some very remarkable and promising uses in stem cell studies.

... we're beginning to see the end of most diseases because stem cells offer treatments, and even cures.

CHAPTER 8

HORMONAL BALANCE MORE ANTI-AGING SECRETS

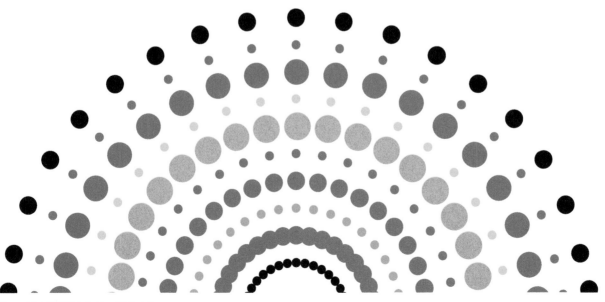

*"If you just set people in motion,
they'll heal themselves"*
GABRIELLE ROTH

BRIEF OVERVIEW OF THE HORMONAL SYSTEM

The endocrine system is one of the major communication networks in the body, consisting of glands that perform specialized tasks by secreting "hormones" or chemical messengers. It sends information via the blood all over the body like a **radio transmitting station**. The pineal and pituitary glands stimulate other endocrine glands to release hormones into the blood stream and, in turn, trigger various responses critical to maintaining homeostasis (such as the thyroid gland to control metabolism, the adrenal glands and the reproductive system to secrete the sex hormones). A prerequisite for any hormone to exert its actions is that it must first bind to specific, high-affinity cellular receptor sites. Hormones secreted by the endocrine glands have powerful and widespread effects in the human body. There are depletions in the hormones with every aspect of aging—bone loss, skin wrinkling and other degenerative conditions. These hormones can become blocked, replaced by estrogen mimickers, altered or modified by our toxic chemical use of products in our air and food. For example, when estrogen and progesterone levels drop, bone density and skin elasticity decline. Low thyroid results in weight gain, fatigue and dry skin.

Endocrine disrupters also referred to as "**gender benders,**" have become rampant in our environment. These are synthetic chemicals that affect the endocrine system as described in detail in the book 'Our Stolen Future'—altering hormonal function. Environmental estrogens or Xeno-estrogens have been the most studied of all the endocrine disrupters. External toxic exposures from various sources (like insecticides, fungicides, plastics, detergents, perfumes that absorb through the skin, birth control pills, hormone replacement therapy) has put our endocrine gland system into confusion.

Modern industrial chemicals and household chemicals have been found to produce Xeno-estrogens or foreign estrogens which are taken up by the estrogen receptor sites in the body. These estrogen-like mimics accumulate in fat tissue such as breasts, ovaries and uterus, creating havoc by interfering with our natural biochemical and hormonal functions. They have been found to unleash a torrent of effects: **reduced sperm production (which plunged worldwide by 50% between 1938 and 1990), cell division, altered sexual behavior, lowered immunity, increased genital deformities, and breast, ovaries, uterine, prostate and testicular cancer.**

The jury is out that these estrogen mimickers are making males more female. **Men are increasingly acquiring female blood characteristics and developing male breasts**—a common condition called **Gynecomastia.** In many animal studies around the world, scientists are finding similar results due to the concentrated Xenoestrogens so pervasive in our environment: emasculated males, male breast growth, decreasing sperm counts, low testosterone and high levels of estrogens in both sexes.

These estrogenic chemicals are found everywhere; affecting animals and humans. They mostly come from the petrochemical industry. Millions of products, including microchips, medicines, synthetic vitamins, clothing, foods, household cleansers, (www.vibrational-cleaning.com) cosmetics, antiperspirants, soaps, toothpaste, herbicides (DDT, dieldrin), pesticides and perfumes either contain or are made from petrochemicals or other man-made synthetics. They're also found in canned foods, plastics, personal care products and food packaging. New research on the long-term effects of these chemicals is constantly being published.

This is not an exhaustive list—there are other sources that are high in xeno-estrogens such as our water, food (dyes, meat sources, dairy products).

WE HAVE BECOME THE TOXIC DUMPSITES! WHAT TO DO?

Step #1 is to **Eliminate** the toxins from your life, from your body, mind and spirit. Toxic accumulations, both physically and emotionally, cause aging and illness.

Step #2 is to **Cleanse**, detoxify or purify the body-mind.

Step #3 is to **Nourish**, revitalize your body-mind and spirit with proper nutrients, quality food and nourishing, loving thoughts.

Before we can truly balance our hormones, the toxic chemicals need to be eliminated and then detoxified. Then we can restore our hormones with the proper nutrients.

ANTI-AGING HORMONES

Researchers have been studying the role of hormones and anti-aging for decades.

Below is a summary of some of the most important hormones to balance.

Pregenenolone

"Of all the hormones in the body, Pregnenolone may be the most important for health and longevity" (D. Gary Young, 2000).

Dr. Gary Young, in his book entitled **Pregnenolone,** describes pregnenolone's many forgotten or ignored virtues. Pregnenolone is a neurosteroid, considered to be a master hormone. It is made in the body from cholesterol produced in the adrenals, the glial cells of the brain and the Schwann cells of the nervous system. It acts as the major precursor or "mother" for all the other naturally occurring steroid hormones like progesterone, (Dehydroepiandrosterone) DHEA, estriol, estradiol, testosterone and many others.

This natural hormone, studied intensely in the 1940s, has been greatly overlooked and suppressed by current medicine. This hormone declines with age. Between the ages of 35 to 75, this hormone drops over 60%. One of the reasons for the drastic decline is given to the use of cholesterol-lowering drugs and low cholesterol diets which contributes to decreased levels of Pregnenolone (remember, it is created from cholesterol). This, in turn, leads to hormonal imbalances linked to accelerated aging, depression, shortened life expectancy and the hastened onset of disease.

Supplemental Pregnenolone is molecularly identical to the Pregnenolone that the body makes naturally. The raw material to create Pregnenolone comes from wild yams (Dioscorea villosa), which are grown in Mexico and other tropical regions throughout the world. Recent studies show Pregnenolone to:

- improve hormonal balance
- enhance memory and cognition
- promote mood elevation and emotional health
- gain proper sleep
- reduce stress
- relieve depression and arthritis
- increase longevity
- reverse wrinkling of the skin and hydrate the skin

Dr. Young concludes in his book that Pregnenolone can be the ideal hormone replacement for both sexes. Due to its precursor function, it endows it as a far safer and effective hormone than by administering any other single hormone alone. Young Living offers this hormone as a capsule. It can be found in a formula called PD 80/20 capsules.

THYROID

Dr. Julian Whitaker reports that an estimated 1 in 5 women over 65 and a significant number of men have low thyroid function. Thyroid conditions are viewed by many alternative health care practitioners as an epidemic problem and more so since Fukishima, Japan, with the extra and continuous leakage of radioactivity in the world! The toxic exposures to substances that inhibit thyroid function are increasing daily in our environment.

Statistics show that nearly the entire U.S. population is deficient in iodine that is essential for the thyroid and according to Dr. Brownstein, Board-Certified family physician, a foremost practitioner of holistic medicine who has specialized in thyroid disorders, says that up to 40% of the population may be suffering from a thyroid disorder and according to reports in the *Life Extension Magazine*—Nearly 74% of normal, "healthy" adults may no longer consume enough iodine.

One of the main reasons is that our diet does not supply enough iodine, including the many commercial brands of table salt. Iodine is essential for metabolic functions and cellular health. It is absolutely vital for the healthy function of our thyroid gland, as Iodine is essential to life and especially crucial for brain development in children, making its deficiency the number one cause of preventable mental retardation worldwide.

Thyroid hormones control our body's metabolism, our internal thermostat, regulating everything from body temperature and heart rate to glucose consumption and even blood lipid levels.

Thyroid deficiencies can manifest as fatigue, **depression**, forgetfulness, weight gain, elevated cholesterol levels, constipation, dry skin, hair loss, goitre and cold hands and feet.

As mentioned earlier, Dr. David Brownstein, who has focused his research on thyroid issues, states that up to 40% of the population may be suffering from a thyroid disorder. (www. drbrownstein.com) Dr. E. Berg in *Healthy Hormones, Healthy Life* points out that there are many people in their 40s to 50s who have secondary thyroid conditions due to endocrine disrupter overload which alters the receptor sites in the thyroid, making the thyroid hormones unavailable.

The best solution to thyroid and endocrine imbalance is to detox these endocrine disrupters as was mentioned earlier. There are a number of products on the market today offered by Dr. Mercola and Dr. Brownstein. Products offered by Young Living, include supplements of Thyromin, Juva Tone, Comfort Tone, Multi Greens, and oil blends of Endo Flex, Purification, Valor, Clarity, Brain Power and single oils of Frankincense, Helichrysum, Myrrh and Myrtle. These are all helpful to optimize the function of the thyroid and help to remove these endocrine disruptor chemicals. Many herbal combinations also assist in detoxing these chemicals—and iodine supplementation along with seaweed may be most helpful.

PINEAL

A major Key to Anti-Aging
The master gland

The most mysterious gland is now being discovered and appreciated as our **anti-aging and most important gland. The pineal gland is part of one of the most significant and least understood systems of our bodies, considered to be the center of our intuition and the "master gland,"** that controls the other endocrine glands. This organ, the size of a grain of rice, lies deep within the human brain at its geometrical center and has been a mystery for nearly two thousand years.

In recent years, findings in neurochemistry and anthropology have given greater credence to the folklore that the pineal gland is the 'third eye', source of 'second sight', 'seat of the soul', or psychic centre within the brain. (see *Vibrational Cleaning* book)

It is a very active organ, having the **second highest blood flow** after the kidneys and equal in volume to the pituitary. The pineal has the highest absorption of phosphorus in the whole body and the *second highest absorption of iodine,* **after the thyroid**. Iodine consumption becomes even more important to the health of the Pineal gland as well as the Thyroid.

No other part of the brain contains so much serotonin or is capable of making melatonin than the Pineal. **Melatonin** has been studied for its effects as an antioxidant, age reversal, and its effects on sleep and insomnia. It is sensitive to stress, electromagnetic fields, light, petro chemicals, pesticides etc. and most notably, fluoride. The pineal strengthens the thymus, fights viruses and rejuvenates the thyroid. It is also a powerful protector against cancer and heart problems, and regulates cycles. Now, what happens when the pineal doesn't or can't produce enough melatonin? This is being found to be the case in many people today, especially those suffering with Alzheimer's.

A new study looked at the intracranial calcifications in the brains of Alzheimer's patients and noticed that the brain's primary structures were negatively affected by calcification, specifically the pineal gland!

Alzheimer's patients showed highly calcified pineal glands, as does two-thirds of the adult population. Alzheimer's disease patients are commonly **deficient in melatonin levels,** likely due to the **inability of their pineal gland to produce** adequate quantities of melatonin. The pineal gland is responsible for regulating melatonin and serotonin. The new findings have postulated a new hypothesis- that **removing calcification from the brain could treat the disease and many others that are now being identified to pineal calcification**.

The International Center for Nutritional Research supports this new hypothesis that calcification of the pineal gland can be causing Alzheimer's disease. In fact, Alzheimer's patients have been observed to have a **higher degree of pineal gland calcification than patients with other types of dementia** and sleep disturbances have been identified as a primary cause of Alzheimer's disease pathogenesis.

Fluoride was shown for the first time to readily accumulate in the human pineal gland.

"Fluoride is likely to cause decreased melatonin production and to have other effects on normal pineal function, which in turn could contribute to a variety of effects in humans" (National Research Council 2006).

Melatonin isn't the only hormone produced in the pineal gland; it also creates a recently discovered substance called **pinoline**. Pinoline is superior to melatonin in aiding DNA replication.

In one experiment (Whitaker, July 2, 2002 – Volume 12, No. 7), Whitaker points out how the pineal glands from young mice were transplanted into old mice and vice versa. The aged mice suddenly had renewed energy and vigor, and lived 12% longer than expected. The young mice with old pineals aged rapidly and died prematurely.

Essential oils have the ability to cross the blood-brain barrier and affect the pineal-pituitary glands and aid in decalcification, along with many other suggestions listed in this guidebook. Vetiver, Cedarwood, Sandalwood, Frankincense, Blue Cypress, Idaho Blue Spruce and Young Living blends called Brain Power, Present Time, Envision, Believe, Magnify Your Purpose and Into the Future are excellent in restoring pineal balance.

Avoidance and minimizing chemical toxins, Fluoride, pesticides, **electromagnetic exposures**—(very damaging to this gland) television, computers, cell phone radiation, microwaves, electrical alarm clocks – to name a few, will help to reduce another insidious toxic pollutant to the pineal. Further details can be obtained from my other books entitled *Vibrational Cleaning* and *Your Right to Know: Vibrational Cleaning Guidebook*.

Edgar Cayce once said: *"Keep the Pineal Gland Operating and You Won't Grow Old —You Will Always be Young."*

DHEA

DHEA (Dehydroepiandrosterone) is produced by the adrenal glands and in the gonads. It is a precursor to testosterone and estrogen. DHEA has been shown to improve erectile dysfunction, libido and sexual satisfaction in older women. It preserves bone density, improves mood, immune function, skin thickness, pigmentation, and hydration. It also increases muscle strength and lean body mass. DHEA levels decrease when stress levels increase. In other words when cortisol production is elevated due to high stress, DHEA is lowered. This is another critical reason to lessen stress levels.

Dr. Neecie Moore reports many studies and uses of DHEA in her book entitled, *Bountiful Health, Boundless Energy, Brilliant Youth: The Facts About DHEA*. Considered to be the "Fountain of Youth" hormone, DHEA accelerates weight loss, aids diabetes, has a significant protective role in cardiovascular disease, aids in menopausal distress, restores hormonal balance, aids in osteoporosis, arthritis, multiple sclerosis, cancer prevention, acts as an antidepressant, and helps with aging and memory. DHEA can be found in Young Living's products, i.e. Corti Stop for women and PD 80/20. Some researchers believe that the combining of small amounts of DHEA with Pregnenolone produces better hormone balance. The above products contain both hormones.

HUMAN GROWTH HORMONE (HGH)

HGH has been studied for its ability to slow the aging process. There is a decreased HGH production with old age. Effects of reduced amounts show as:

- fine lines and wrinkles
- sagging, baggy skin
- failing sexual performance
- poor memory
- thinning, graying hair
- failing eyesight
- decreased mobility
- cardiovascular problems

- weight management
- blood pressure problems

There have been well over 20,000 studies, abstracts and reports documenting the many truly wonderful benefits of HGH:

- sharper vision and improved hearing
- enhanced memory
- pain-free movement
- greater resistance vs. illness
- increased sexual potency
- diminished wrinkles, much better skin elasticity, tone and feel
- hair re-growth
- cholesterol, blood pressure improvements

In one study of 36 people, scientists (Jamieson & Dorman) evaluated the effectiveness of HGH in the form of symbiotropin. IGF-1 levels were measured as an indicator for the growth hormone over a 12 week period. IGF-1 levels increased by 30%, reporting many overall physical, mental and emotional improvements. A summary of improvements after 12 weeks for the hair and skin are given below:

- skin texture – 47%
- skin thickness – 32%
- skin elasticity – 26%
- wrinkle disappearance – 37%
- new hair growth – 47%

Longevity Blend—is considered as one of the world's strongest antioxidant supplements due to containing Thyme, Clove, and Frankincense and Orange oils.

Dr. Radwan Farag was among the first to show in vitro how selected essential oils were able to significantly slow the oxidation of unsaturated fatty oils, particularly the essential oils of Thyme, Clove, Rosemary and Sage. They are best to be taken as food supplements. Semmelweis University of Medicine in 1993 documented these remarkable antioxidant effects. Results from their studies were phenomenal. Researchers found that daily **life-long feeding of Thyme and Clove oils** to laboratory animals preserved key antioxidant levels in the liver, kidneys, heart and brain. In effect, the essential oils were slowing, and even reversing, the aging process. In another study, these same essential oils **restored DHA levels in the eyes** to levels found in much younger subjects. The brain is another organ where omega-3 fatty acids like DHA (decosahexaenoic acid) are essential to health. **Thyme oil dramatically slowed age-related DHA and PUFA (polyunsaturated fatty acids) degradation in the brain.** In other words, the essential oil of **Thyme** was able to partially

prevent brain aging by protecting its essential fatty acids. Thyme oil, steam-distilled from thymus vulgaris, has been found to slow and reverse aging.

Clove Oil – research showed potent antioxidant-boosting properties plus anti-carcinogenic agents. Clove oil is the highest antioxidant essential oil – 400 times more potent than the highest antioxidant food that has been identified the Ningxia wolfberries. An **ounce of Clove oil** has the antioxidant capacity of **450 pounds of carrots, 120 quarts of blueberries or 48 gallons of beet juice** (Dr. David Stewart, *Healing Oils of the Bible* 2002:18). One researcher found that 5% eugenol in Clove oil protected test animals against mutagenic and cancer-causing effects of the chemical benzopyrene. **Orange, Lemon and Peppermint oils** were shown to retard the formation of tumors and reduce the incidence of cancer. The Longevity Blend is available in gel caps containing Thyme, Clove and Orange and Frankincense essential oils.

Frankincense Oil (Boswellia carteri) has a sweet, warm, balsamic aroma that is stimulating and elevating to the mind. There has been a great amount of research as this oil is known for its benefits for visualizing, improving one's spiritual connection and centering. It has comforting properties that help focus the mind and overcome stress and despair. Frankincense is considered as one of the holy anointing oils in the Middle East, where it has been used in religious ceremonies for thousands of years. Frankincense is also a valuable ingredient in skin care products for aging and dry skin and used for thousands of years for regeneration of healthy cells. The ancient Egyptians used it in rejuvenation face masks. More recently, it has been used in European and American hospitals and is the subject of substantial research.

"It was known to treat every conceivable ill known to man." When ingested as a supplement, it helps to boost health and is therefore considered a tonic. It benefits many systems such as the respiratory, digestive, nervous and excretory systems. It aids the absorption of nutrients into the body. It also strengthens the immune system helps regulate estrogen production and delayed menstruation.

- Helps PMS symptoms and pain.
- Relieves cough and phlegm, bronchitis, and congestion
- Improves digestion and alleviates gas, abnormal sweating, uneasiness, and indigestion and is helpful to detox the body.

Frankincense Oil has many virtues and this addition in the Longevity Blend certainly adds more power to heightening the benefits.

ANOTHER AGE ACCELERATOR—ADRENAL BURN-OUT

Cortisol is produced by the body during times of stress or Adrenal exhaustion. Cortisol is referred to as the "death hormone" as high amounts prevent other important hormones to be produced such as HGH, estrogen, testosterone and DHEA (see section on anti-aging hormones). The adrenals are often referred to as **our 'stress buffer' and they are crucial in responding to the stresses in our environment.** It's important to 'reboot' our adrenals and reclaim our energy source that is vital for health and longevity.

CortiStop is a product produced by Young Living Company to help women reduce their cortisol production. This helps the body to function in a healthier state.

Dr David Stewart points out how longevity was common in the early Old Testament days. The fifth chapter of Genesis tells about Adam, who lived 930 years, and Methuselah, who lived 969. Essential oils may have played a role in their virile and vigorous long lives.

Some essential oil suggestions for adrenal support are: Rosemary, Nutmeg, Clove, Idaho Balsam Fir, Frankincense, Lavender and the blends: Endo Flex, En-R-Gee, Common Sense and Stress Away.

Add Ho Shu Wu, Holy Basil and Green tea to boost the adrenals.

There are more Ways to help the Adrenals, Liver and kidneys with a Petrochemical detox.

Another blend for **Petrochemical detox—**Preparation: Add 10 drops of Ledum essential oil into a full bottle of Citrus Fresh essential oil blend.

1. Take 20 drops of Grapefruit essential oil in a capsule before retiring for one week.

2. Apply the Citrus Fresh oil combination over the fat areas and over liver/gallbladder area before retiring.

Drink lots of water during the week to help flush the chemical residues. Eat lightly, preferably raw and green for the week.

FORMALDEHYDE BUILD-UP often from perfumes, plastics, medications, building materials, off gassing of new materials, fabrics, carpets, etc. These are absorbed from the many products that have used this chemical.

Use Purification oil (Citronella, Lemongrass, Lavandin, Rosemary, Melaleuca and Mrytle) to help remove build-up.

Apply on feet; over liver and kidneys; on brain stem, along with detoxifying your liver with herbal and essential oil combinations.

DANGERS OF SYNTHETIC HORMONE REPLACEMENT

Many reports over the years have surfaced about the dangers in using synthetic hormone replacement therapy. An article in TIME, July 15, 2002, raises again the safety issue: "Not only did HRT fail to reduce the risk of heart attacks and strokes, it significantly increased the incidence of blood clots and gall bladder disease." The study was published in the Journal of the American Medical Association – a seven-year study.

A follow up report in TIME, July 22, 2002, reported again the "Truth About Hormones." A large federally funded clinical trial, part of a group of studies called the Women's Health Initiative, has definitely shown that the synthetic hormones in question – estrogen and progestin – are not the age-defying wonder drugs everyone thought they were. It was shown that taking these hormones for more than a few years actually increases a woman's risk of developing potentially deadly cardiovascular problems and invasive breast cancer. **The findings were so striking – the study was stopped 3 years short of its schedule.**

SUMMARY OF HORMONAL DISRUPTION

CAUSE	EFFECT
1. Excess blood glucose from sugar, carbohydrates, allergenic foods	Advances aging
2. Excess insulin levels due to sugar and refined carbohydrates	Interferes with hormones (HGH) and glucagons, producing more stress hormone – cortisol
3. Excess cortisol levels	High stress, wears out all body systems; thymus gland is very sensitive to high cortisol, weakening the immune function.
4. Excess free radicals (from the petrochemicals, pesticides, toiletries etc.)	Accelerates the aging process; fewer free radicals – longer life. Overeating and high caloric intake produces free radicals as well as the chemicals, pollutants and toxins previously discussed in other chapters.

CHAPTER 9

YOUTH FOODS AND NECESSARY FATS

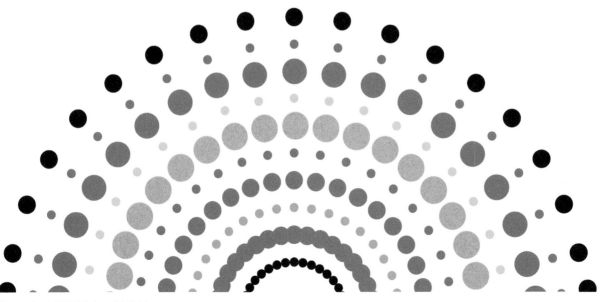

"Food can Heal and Renew.
Food can be your anti-aging medicine."
DEEPAK CHOPRA

Sound nutritional habits to nurture your body are essential for rejuvenating your mind and body and to acquiring beautiful skin. To reverse aging through eating wisely is not difficult—it is a matter of attention, focus and commitment. You are what you eat!

An anti-inflammatory diet and super-antioxidant diet is recommended. One that is high in fruits and vegetables.

- **Avoid sugar**, even raw sugar, as it still creates Glycosylation of the skin where skin becomes inflexible and prone to discolor. Low carbohydrates that are high on the Glycemic index include **bananas, carrots, corn, mangoes, papaya, potatoes and rice.**
- **Avoid processed and packaged foods** laden with chemical additives.
- **Avoid dairy** products; the most digestible is organic goat's milk.
- **Reduce intake of animal fat.** Increase cold water fishes and lean fowl.
- **Chew your food** well, until it becomes a liquid. This helps to digest your food. Savor the flavors.
- For dry skin conditions, increase your intake of essential fatty acids.
- Begin your meals with a blessing or thoughts of gratitude. Prepare your mind and body to receive your food.
- Consume foods that include the six flavors (sweet, sour, salty, pungent, bitter, astringent) throughout the day.
- Buy organically grown foods as much as possible. Eat a diet high in protein (fish, chicken, turkey, legumes, nuts), moderate carbohydrates (whole meal sprouted grain bread, whole grain cereals- better grain **Einkorn**) and unsaturated fats (use cold pressed vegetable oils; extra virgin olive oil, coconut oil, hemp oil, sesame or walnut oils).
- Eat fermented foods that support healthy gut function

- Eat plenty of fruits and vegetables; more plant foods with high antioxidant levels like berries, turmeric, green leafy vegetables; well scrubbed, raw in salads or lightly cooked. Sweeten foods sparingly with agave, Stevia extract or Stevia select. All have a low Glycemic index, ideal for anyone with diabetes or hypoglycemia.
- Make sure to get plenty of Vit D—take a supplement if your blood levels are low, vitamin B12, folic acid, magnesium and zinc and omega 3 which all have a beneficial impact on reducing stress levels and impacting telomere length
- Eat grapes, cacao and cacao butter which contain resveratrol to help repair DNA from free radical damage and to de-stress
- Consume more berries esp. blueberries. (higher antioxidants)
- Drink Matcha green tea or Reishi tea
- Find ways to exercise with bursts of high intensity. Exercise is one of the biggest ways to change telomere length.
- Find a relaxation activity everyday—music, yoga, hugs, laughter, meditation, dance, walks, whatever lifts your mood.
- Surround your space with essential oils to uplift your mood –Citrus Fresh, Cedarwood, lavender, orange, lemon, lime, Present Time

EAT YOUR VEGGIES!

An international study on eating patterns and skin aging found that dark and fair-skinned people who ate plenty of wholesome foods (declined sugary foods) were less prone to wrinkling. Researchers found consistent results worldwide, be it sun-drenched Australia or sun-deprived Sweden.

Some of the skin-smoothing foods were green leafy vegetables, beans, olive oil and nuts. People who ate more of the foods that are universally recommended for good health had smoother skin. The authors speculate that the foods offered skin protection due to their high levels of antioxidants. (Journal of the American College of Nutrition, 2001: 20:71 – 80)

BERRIES ARE BERRY BERRY NICE

Doctors are now prescribing berries due to their high antioxidant levels. They are also high in flavanoids. So eat your berries as they strengthen connective tissue. Ningxia Red—a Young Living berry Juice, according to ORAC, is one of the highest in antioxidants.

Scientists at USDA have developed a rating scale that measures antioxidant content of plant foods called ORAC—oxygen radical absorbent capacity. See findings—the best in anti-aging foods. ***Chinese wolfberries are the highest scoring antioxidant food in the world.***

LOW GLYCEMIC FOODS INCLUDE:	HIGH ANTI-OXIDANT FOODS:
• Asparagus	• Avocado
• Broccoli	• Berries—especially wolfberries
• Blueberries	• Cantaloupe
• Cabbage	• Salmon
• Cantaloupe	• Tomatoes
• Citrus	• Squash
• Kiwi	• Spinach/kale
• Leafy greens	• Plums
• Peaches	
• Pears	
• Plums	
• Spinach	
• Non-starch vegetables	

THE ORAC SCALE

A new test developed by USDA researchers at Tuft University in Boston, Mass., has been able to identify the highest known antioxidant in foods. Known as ORAC (oxygen radical absorbent capacity), this test is the first of its kind to measure both time and degree of free-radical inhibition. See table following.

ESSENTIAL OILS	ANTIOXIDANT CAPACITY*	FOODS	ANTIOXIDANT CAPACITY**
Clove	10,786,875	Ningxia Wolfberry	25,300
Cinnamon Bark	103,448	Blueberries	2,400
Thyme	159,590	Kale	1,770
Oregano	153,007	Strawberries	1,540
Mountain Savory	113,071	Spinach	1,260
Cistus	38,648	Raspberries	1,220
Eucalyptus globulus	24,157	Brussels Sprouts	980
Orange	18,898	Plums	949
Lemongrass	17,765		
Helichrysum	17,430	Broccoli florets	890
Ravensara	8,927	Beets	840
Lemon	6,125	Oranges	750
Spearmint	5,398	Red grapes	739
Lavender	3,669	Red bell peppers	710
Rosemary CT cineole	3,309	Cherries	670
Juniper	2,517	Yellow corn	400
Roman Chamomile	2,446	Eggplant	390
Sandalwood	1,655	Carrots	210

* Antioxidant capacity for oils is estimated by Ferric Reducing Power and is expressed as micromole Trolox Equivalents (TE) per liter.

** For foods, it is expressed as TE per 100 grams. (from Essential Oils Desk Reference, page 415)

The USDA recommends that you eat at least 3,000 ORAC units a day.

HEALTH EFFECTS OF VIRGIN OLIVE OIL

Excerpt from **Fats that Heal and Fats that Kill**, Udo Erasmus.

Studies carried out with virgin olive oil show that it helps membrane development, cell formation and cell differentiation! Virgin olive oil improves brain maturation and brain function when there is a deficiency of EFA (essential fatty acids). Olive oil is rich in vital antioxidants—containing antioxidant polyphenol (including a substance known as oleocanthal which has anti-inflammatory properties) plus tyrosol and squalene, essential amino acids and flavonoids. Skin aging, as well as general body aging, seems to be closely tied to the inflammatory process. Olive Oil is also rich in Omega components such as Omega 9, Vitamin A, Vitamin K, traces of Vitamin C and Vitamin E which is, in and of itself, another antioxidant.

Due to these all powerful anti-aging agents rubbing Olive Oil into your skin on a daily basis can slow down the aging process and help to maintain a healthy vibrant glowing skin. Use Olive Oil in therapeutic massage.

In patients with peripheral artery disease on fat-lowering diets, a switch from corn oil (refined) to virgin olive oil (unrefined) for six months resulted in significantly decreased "bad" LDL cholesterol and significantly increased "good" HDL cholesterol. In other words, virgin olive oil performed much better than corn oil for these patients.

Monounsaturated fatty acid-rich virgin olive oil has also been shown to reduce the production of cholesterol gallstones and to favor bile secretion, which improves elimination of the toxic end-products of liver detoxification and improves digestion of fats.

The minor components in olive oil also have some specific beneficial effects:

- Beta-sitosterol lowers high cholesterol levels.
- Triterpenic acids have healing and anti-inflammatory effects.
- Caffeic and gallic acids stimulate the flow of bile.
- Gallic acid also inhibits lactic dehydrogenase activity in the liver (sign of liver malfunction).
- Phenolic compounds protect against peroxidation of fatty acids and cholesterol.
- 2-phenylethanol stimulates the production of fat-digesting enzymes in the pancreas.
- Triterpenic acids found only in olive oil also stimulate these pancreatic enzymes.
- Cycloartenol, stored in the liver, lowers the amount of circulating cholesterol and increase bile excretion.

A combination of 2-phenylethanol and triterpenic acids slows down cholesterol digestion and decreases cholesterol absorption from foods.

The virtues of olive oil for anti-aging have been known for thousands of years. Jeanne Louise Calment, a French super centenarian who lived to the age of 122 years and 164 days, based her long life on the consumption and usage of olive oil. In ancient times the Olive was revered for its longevity, life sustaining powers and skin regenerating properties.

Due to the olive tree's ability to live for thousands of years, people believed that the qualities inherent in Olive trees for longevity were contained in the fruit and oil of the tree. They believed that that these qualities could be passed on to the peoples of the Earth who consumed the Olives along with the precious oil.

The great physicians of antiquity, Hippocrates, Diocles and Galen all knew the skin rejuvenating powers of olive oil. They praised and utilized olive oil in their medical practices and ointments. Galen, for example, who is credited with the invention of the cold cream used Olive Oil, Beeswax and Rosewater in the 2nd century AD as a moisturizer.

GreenMedInfo.com presents a database of research on the properties of Olive Oil that contribute to its' tremendous ability in healing various health conditions and repairing our skin.

EPA AND DHA OILS

EPA and DHA are normal constituents in our cells. They are especially abundant in brain cells, nerve relay stations, visual receptors, adrenal glands and sex glands – the most biochemically active tissues in our body. Both can be produced by healthy cells from essential 3-fatty acid, alpha-linolenic acids (LNA) this is found abundantly in oils from flax, black currant and several other seeds. However, degenerative conditions may impair our body's ability to make EPA and DHA from LNA.

Cold-water fish also contain EPA and DHA. They make it from the brown and red algae they digest.

Here are some of the benefits from EPA and DHA oils:

- Platelets: EPA and DHA keep our platelets from getting too sticky, resulting in less likelihood of clots that can cause heart attack or stroke.
- Arteries: EPA and DHA help repair the arteries, resulting in less arteriosclerosis and more open arteries.
- Blood triglycerides: EPA and DHA can lower triglycerides and cholesterol level, which is important for lowering high blood pressure and preventing arteriosclerosis, heart and kidney failure, stroke and heart attack.
- Hormone effects: From EPA, our body makes PG3 prostaglandins and leukotrienes, which help prevent strokes, heart attack and other problems that involve blood clot formation, such as pulmonary embolism and cardiovascular complications accompanying diabetes.

- Cancer: In some animal studies, fish oils inhibit growth and metastasis of tumors. Interesting, negative results with fish oils in cancer treatments are likely due to poor product quality or rancid oils.
- Blood pressure: EPA lowers elevated blood pressure.

Black currant fruits and juice, known to be rich in a specific flavanoids called anthocyanoside, are commonly consumed in many parts of the world and contains gamma linolenic acid (GLA). GLA can help in a number of different circumstances including eczema, rheumatoid arthritis, premenstrual syndrome, and attention deficit disorder.

GLA helps strengthen hair and decreases breakage by helping to decrease the effect of imbalanced hormonal effects, which weaken and thin your hair. A typical supplemental dose is 500mg twice a day.

MORE ON OMEGA 3S—CHIA SEEDS

The new rave in omega 3's is Chia seeds as it has been found to have the highest level of Omega 3s in any plant. We no longer need to rely on fish oils as the only source for Omega 3s. We can consume all of our Omega 3s from green leafy vegetables, legumes, flax seeds, **Chia seeds** or walnuts, besides highly purified fish oil supplements, or algae-sourced Omega-3 supplements as mentioned earlier in this chapter.

Chia Seeds in particular have been found to be:

- **High in Omega 3s**. Chia seeds are the richest botanical source of omega-3 fatty acids found in nature and of any plant including flax seed. This is in the form of alpha-linolenic acid –which has cardio protective & neuro protective benefits of ALA. It is also effective in countering inflammation and has a beneficial effect on autoimmune diseases.
- The fatty acids encourage the formation of collagen and elastin, which support skin structure and helps maintain moisture levels. (so Chia is great to use as a mask—see section under masks)
- Chia seeds are high in fiber—considered to be the highest whole-food source of fiber.
- Easy storage as it doesn't need refrigeration like flaxseed. It's so rich in anti-oxidants (chlorogenic acid, caffeic acid, myricetin, quercetin and flavonols).
- Chia seeds also contain a number of nutrients: protein, calcium, phosphorus, magnesium, manganese, copper, niacin and zinc.
- Chia is easy to add to food as it is tasteless. Mix in oatmeal, yogurt, baked goods, or smoothies. Sprinkle on salads.

- Chia seeds are high in alpha-lipoic acids. Alpha-lipoic acid is known to help minimize fine lines, wrinkles and enlarged pores, while encouraging healthy cellular function and increasing radiance in the skin.

The coolest thing about Chia seeds is that when you add liquid they expand, it's like a magic show!!!

SEA BUCKTHORN BERRY OIL CAPSULES

Sea Buckthorn (Hippophae rhamnoides L.) is an interesting berry that doesn't necessarily grow beside the sea. It is native from north-western Europe, through central Asia as well as northern China. It is **believed to have originated from the Himalayas, but was also used by European cultures and the ancient Greeks as far back as 12 B.C. to treat various health issues. It appears in the ancient Tibetan texts, is mentioned in the Indian Materia Medica, early Chinese formularies and ancient Greek mythology.** It is renowned in Ayurvedic medicine as far back as 5000 BC.

Sea buckthorn is known in Tibet, Russia, Mongolia, and China to help relieve cough, promote blood circulation, aid digestion, and alleviate pain. It was used for centuries as a food and for its pharmaceutical properties. (Mercola)

Anecdotal reports indicate sea buckthorn was used in ancient times to:

- Lower fevers, reduce inflammation, counteract toxicity and abscesses and clean the lungs.
- Treat colds and coughs.
- Treat tumours and growths, especially of the stomach and the oesophagus.

Sea Buckthorn is rich in many essential nutrients that have strong antioxidant activity and anti-inflammatory properties. It contains over 190 nutrients and Phytonutrients, including vitamin C, which is 12 times higher than that of an orange. It contains three times more vitamin A than carrots, and four times more superoxide dismutase (SOD), than ginseng, an important enzyme that helps prevent free radical damage. No wonder it's considered a superfood.

The oil is extracted from both the fruit and from the seed. It is rich in vitamin E, carotenoids, phytosterols (that helps to reduce redness and help heal mucous membranes) plus essential fatty acids. It is extraordinarily rich, perfectly balanced and the only plant source in omega 3, 6, 7 and 9 oils aiding healing from the inside out.

Topical application of sea buckthorn oil balances and harmonizes the lipid layers of the skin and is a great cleanser and exfoliator. It is beneficial for all skin types and has been reported for skin therapy including sun, heat, chemical and radiation burns, eczema and poorly healing wounds (Mercola, Chatelaine) .

It is known to promote excellent skin health and anti-aging-hydration, elasticity and skin regeneration. It also helps with weight management and helps to prevent dementia/ Alzheimer due to its B12 content and omega 3s.

Sea buckthorn oil is generally safe for most adults but not for people with diseases of the intestines, kidney and liver and for children under the age of 12.

COENZYME Q-10

Our bodies naturally make CoQ10 (also known as ubiquinone), a nutrient necessary for basic cell function. It enters the mitochondria (our cells' "energy centers"), where it helps transform fats and sugars into energy. As we age, CoQ10 levels naturally decline.

Test-tube and animal studies show that CoQ10 acts as a protective antioxidant in mito-chondrial membranes and may prevent cognitive decline.

When taken with other antioxidants—selenium and vitamins C and E—CoQ10 may also improve arterial elasticity, making you less vulnerable to the hardening of the arteries that leads to heart disease, according to a 2010 study published in Nutrition & Metabolism.

Recommended dose: Take 30–200 mg per day, according to the University of Maryland's program in complementary medicine.

RESVERATROL

Resveratrol has gained a lot of attention in the anti-aging department in the last few years as well as in combating diseases. Early research, mostly done in test tubes and in animals, suggests that resveratrol might help protect the body against a number of diseases, such as heart disease, diabetes, cancer, and Alzheimer's.

Known as the "red wine" chemical, resveratrol is a polyphenol found in the skin of grapes and berries. A Mayo Clinic article points out that some research shows that resveratrol could be linked to a reduced risk of inflammation and blood clotting, both of which can lead to heart disease. Other animal research has found that mice given resveratrol sur-vived longer than two other groups, one fed a standard diet, the other a high-calorie diet.

As more research is explored in this area—it will be interesting to see how much this nutrient will have in anti-aging. Increasing your berry consumption will certainly be beneficial.

TURMERIC

Turmeric is another spice—food that has been gaining more reviews and popularity in the West for many of its benefits. It's an ancient Indian spice that gives curry its flavor and yellow color to Indian dishes or as an Ayurveda or Chinese medicine.

It is known for its anti-inflammatory and protective antioxidant properties. It is a member of the ginger family, and has been found to help shield against a variety of age-related conditions.

It is well known in India as a good way to improve skin health and for many other health problems. Turmeric has a long history in being used as an essential part of any beauty treatment in many parts of India and highly used in Indian wedding rituals that are applied to both the bridegroom and bride. The paste or face mask is used to treat various skin conditions like stretch marks, wrinkles, pigmentation, acne, blemishes, dark spots, eczema and rosacea etc.

Due to Turmeric's anti-inflammatory and anti-oxidant properties it is effective in treating these skin conditions For individuals with eczema, applying a facial mask can reduce inflammation and red-ness. For rosacea individuals turmeric masks can reduce the tiny pimples and redness that this skin condition causes. Turmeric is also known to have many beauty benefits such as healing dry skin, slowing down the aging process and making the skin supple.

A University of California, Irvine study in 2010 found that turmeric's active ingredient, curcumin, extended the lifespan of fruit flies by up to 20%. Another study at the University of Arizona in 2010 suggested that the extract can help prevent arthritis and bone loss in aging women. Many more internet sites are touting Turmeric's many benefits. According to a 2006 study in Singapore, older adults who reported having curry "occasionally" scored better on mental health tests than those who "never or rarely" consumed the dish.

So far from human studies it is recommended to use 1-gram supplement daily.

CUCUMBER

Is considered to be a great detoxifying fruit—by helping to flush the kidneys, cleanse the bowels, aid digestive health. It is high in minerals such as calcium, magnesium, sulfur, silica found in the skin, and vitamins E and C. It even contains an enzyme that dissolves tapeworms.

WATERMELON

This fruit is best to be eaten on its own. Very helpful to flush the kidneys, help flush the digestive system, is alkalizing and very high in silica.

MULTIVITAMINS

Most people are aware that a daily multivitamin can make up for nutritional deficits in your diet. Research on vitamin-mineral intake also suggests that it could lead to a longer life.

According to a 2009 National Institutes of Health study, women who took multivitamins regularly had longer Telomeres, (these are the protective caps at the end of chromosomes that grow shorter with age, as discussed earlier in Chapter 4). Longer telomeres are associated with youth and health,whereas, shorter ones with aging and disease. The study also found a link between longer telomeres and higher intakes of vitamins C and E from food and also Vitamin D from another 2007 study at the London School of Medicine.

AGILEASE™

A proprietary combination by Young Living.

A new recent product was created and then introduced to the market in June, 2016 for middle-aged and elderly people as well as athletes to support normal bone and joint health. It is called **Agilease (a proprietary combination by Young Living)**.

AgilEase is an organic dietary supplement that helps users to ease joint discomfort, improve joint flexibility and mobility, as well as restoring joint and cartilage health.

The product contains very unique and powerful ingredients such as frankincense resin powder, UC-II undenatured collagen, hyaluronic acid, calcium fructoborate, and a specially formulated proprietary essential oil blend of Wintergreen, Copaiba, Clove, and Northern Lights Black Spruce—oils that are known for their joint health benefits.

All Ingredients: Frankincense resin powder (Boswellia sacra), calcium fructoborate (from plant minerals), Tumeric rhizome extract (Curcuma longa), Piperine from Black Pepper whole fruit extract (Piper nigrum), Collagen type II (chicken sternum extract), Glucosamine sulfate, Hyaluraunic acid (as sodium hyaluronate), Wintergreen leaf essential oil (Gaultheria procumbens), Copaiba oleoresin wood essential oil (Copaifera officinalis), Northern Lights Black Spruce whole tree oil (Picea mariana) and clove.

THE ESSENTIAL OILS INCLUDE:

Wintergreen Essential Oil (Gaultheria procumbens) which contains 85–99% of methyl salicylate the same active ingredient found in aspirin. It is beneficial for soothing head tension and muscles after exercising or injuries.

Balsam Fir Essential Oil (Abies balsamea) known for use for muscular aches and pains, soothes and rejuvenates body and mind and in supporting respiratory function.

Clove Essential Oil (Syzygium aromaticum) is the highest ranked known antioxidant. It helps to boost immunity and promote oral health.

Northern Lights Black Spruce (Picea mariana) helps improve the appearance of dry skin or to help maintain the appearance of healthy-looking skin. it is also known for its joint health benefits.

ADVANTAGES OF STRENGTH TRAINING AND REVERSING AGING

Movement is essential to an anti-aging program. By not exercising, we increase our risk for heart disease, high blood pressure, diabetes, arthritis and cancer. In one study where healthy men were inactive (bed rest) for three weeks, their measurements of cardiovascular fitness deteriorated by almost twenty years of aging (Chopra, 2001). Dr. Gary Young presents latest research in his book *A New Route to Robust Health* on how strength training increases resilience, strength, health, joint pain and the lowering of blood pressure. He particularly points out how human growth hormone is boosted through resistance training. The amazing results show that the *"activity of lifting weight at just 70% of lifting capacity resulted in tripling of growth hormone levels in the body."* I have pointed out earlier in this book the importance of growth hormones for reversing signs of aging. Some of the other benefits Dr. Young points out are: HGH reshapes physical contours, burns fat and builds muscle, boosts immunity, increases energy and strengthens the heart.

A study done by Dr. Nelson and her colleagues at Tufts University found that 20 women who were monitored over a year doing a strength-training program some time after menopause completely transformed their bodies inside and out. The anti-aging benefits include: thinner physique, higher metabolism, increased strength, more energy, improved mood, added bone and better balance (***Growing Younger*** 2002, by Doherty, Tine Prevention Editors).

Strength training in itself produces a powerful rise in growth hormone which obviously is an important step to add to a youthful program. Exercise is also important for the skin, as it increases the circulation of blood to the skin, delivering the necessary nutrients and disposing the wastes.

ANOTHER AGE SAVER—GET YOUR BEAUTY SLEEP

Dr. Whitaker points out that when you don't get enough sleep, the face looks tired. During sleep, the pituitary gland releases growth hormone and other growth factors that stimulate the production of new collagen—helping to repair and renew the cells.

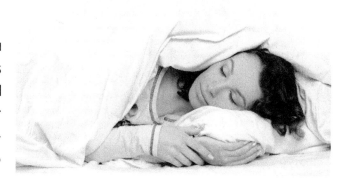

Dr. Young points out that the growth hormone is secreted the most from 11:00 p.m. to 1:00 a.m., and stresses the importance of sleep for health and longevity. Also, the skin around the eyes loses its elasticity and moisture content when one does not get enough sleep.

Dr. Eve Van Cauter, a University of Chicago researcher, found that not having enough sleep robbed people of their health. (Published in Lancet, 1999) In his ground breaking study, healthy young men went through a sleep deprivation program over a three-week period. During the second week where the men had only four hours of sleep, blood samples showed impaired glucose tolerance resulting in the central nervous system becoming more active. In one week, these healthy men were in a pre-diabetic state. Dr. Cauter states that lack of sleep decreases secretion of HGH—growth hormone and accelerates excessive fat gain—partly responsible for rise in obesity; elevates the stress hormone cortisol and diminished melatonin sleep hormone.

Dr. Chopra emphasizes the importance of experiencing deep rest in body and mind. He recommends eight hours of sleep between 10 p.m. and 6 a.m. He also recommends the practice of meditation. Studies have shown that people who practice meditation have DHEA hormone levels higher than in people who do not. Meditation helps one to quiet the mind and experience the restful response.

"Restful sleep accelerates healing,
minimizes entropy; and enlivens renewal."
CHOPRA, 2011

BREATHING AND RELAXING

Many today are quite familiar with the advances that Yogic traditions have been teaching us for thousands of years. The importance of the breath is one that is taught in many healing practices along with meditation. Mastering healthy breathing techniques can transform our life and well-being.

Dr. Andrew Weil is a world-renowned pioneer and leader in the field of integrative medicine, often referred to as the father of Integrative Medicine. He had this to say about breathing: *"If I had to limit my advice on healthier living to just one tip, it would be simply to learn how to breathe correctly. From my own experience and from working with patients, I have come to believe that proper breathing is the master key to good health."*

Studies analysing people's breathing patterns found that they habitually breathe high up in their chest which in effect, puts stress on their heart and the nervous system. **The average adult is breathing 12,000 to 25,000 breaths per day.** By breathing properly and optimally, we enact the full expansion of the lungs and their ability to efficiently deliver Life Force into the body.

An interesting finding from a 5,200-person clinical study group observed over a 30-year span found that **the way a person breathes is the primary measure of potential life span.** (From Framingham study) What has been determined is that the average person reaches peak respiratory function and lung capacity in their mid 20s. As people age they lose between 9% and 25% of respiratory capacity for every decade of their life! **So take a deep breath and make it a lifestyle habit!**

THE POWER OF THE MIND IN ANTI-AGING

The 'new biology' has revolutionized scientific thinking when it was shown that our minds control **our genetic expression. Dr. Bruce Lipton's breakthrough discovery in quantum biology clearly showed how DNA is more influenced by our environment. In other words, our cells and our DNA are more influenced by our thoughts, our beliefs and our imagination than anything else around us.**

Can meditation and mindfulness slow down the aging process? Apparently from recent research in mindfulness meditation, by Drs. Epel and Blackburn, they have found that it does. The answer is, absolutely, YES!

Meditators and those who use mindfulness techniques are slowing down their aging by lengthening their telomeres.

SUMMARY OF LIFE-LONGEVITY PROMOTERS

- Daily exercise or some form of movement
- Healthy eating- organic foods
- Healthy relationships
- Healthy, non-toxic, `vibrational` home environment
- Doing things you love
- Avoiding environmental & chemical toxins
- Adequate water intake
- Not smoking
- Deep breathing practices and relaxation
- Beauty sleep
- Mindfulness and meditation
- Visualization practices
- Anti-aging supplements
- Hormonal balance
- Positive attitude
- Organic facial creams — with essential oils

CHAPTER 10

BENEFITS OF ESSENTIAL OILS

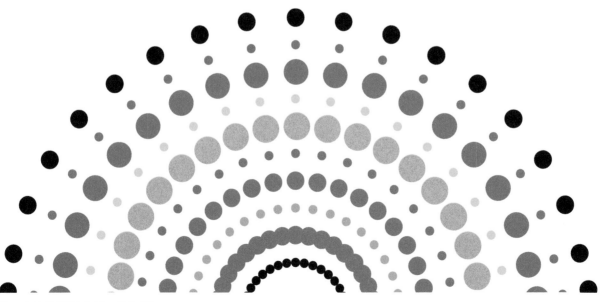

"Cellular regeneration is the key to youthful skin and essential oils provide a way of doing this."
VALERIE ANN WORWOOD

AVOID LETHAL INJECTIONS!

As we've seen earlier, Botox injections are the most popular cosmetic procedure in the U.S. Approximately 1.6 million Americans get their Botox shots each year. Health Sciences Institute reports a very disturbing trend: how women are having "Botox" parties instead of Tupperware or bridge parties. They invite friends to have the poison injected where they have wrinkles, all while munching on chips and salsa.

A better idea, instead of getting shot up with a poison and paralyzing parts of your face, is to use these nurturing beauty benefits of essential oils.

Have a "Scents-able Saving Face Party" instead!

The essential oils described below have many applications and features. This is by no Means a complete Catalog of their properties—only a focused sketch is given specifically for the skin.

Basil (Ocimum basilicum)
Code: O, N
- Stimulates circulation
- Enlivens dull-looking skin
- Improves skin tone
- Gives complexion a rosy glow
- Controls acne
- Adds luster to dull hair
- Excellent nerve tonic – relaxing and uplifting

CODE (FOR SKIN TYPE):

D – Dry

N – Normal

O – Oily

W – Wrinkles

M – Mature skin

Bergamot (Citrus bergamia)
Code: O, M

- Widely cultivated in the Southern part of Italy, specifically in Reggio di Calabria and Sicily and Morocco
- Used in the Middle East for hundreds of years for skin conditions associated with an oily complexion.
- Used in Earl Grey Tea and used in the first genuine eau de cologne
- It's known to provide calming benefits,
- Hormonal support,
- Antidepressant, ease anxiety, depression, and is mood-lifting
- Great natural, chemical-free mosquito repellant,
- Eases insect-bites,
- Use as deodorant and relaxing massage oil.
- Bergamot speeds up the healing process for Herpes cold sores, mouth ulcers, viral infections– and it has a similar antibacterial effect on shingles and chickenpox, which are also caused by the varicella zoster virus from herpes
- Prevent and improve Fungal Skin infections –Italian researchers have proven bergamot essential oil's amazing antifungal, topical properties for Candida fungus strains published in the Journal of Antimicrobial Chemotherapy.

Word of Caution: Similar to all citrus oils, avoid them if basking in the sun or any sun exposure: bergamot oil may induce photosensitivity (oversensitivity to the sun) and may lead to extreme sunburn and other complications due to its bergamottin and bergapten content, which absorbs ultraviolet light.

Blue Cypress (Callitris intartropica)
Code: N

- Antiseptic, antiviral, antitumoral
- Regulates excessive oiliness of the skin or scalp
- Reduces inflammation and blemishes
- Helpful for stress, depression, insomnia

Carrot Seed (Daucus carota)
Code: D, M, W, O

Carrot seed oil is distilled from the tiny, dry seeds of the wild carrot plant commonly known as Queen Anne 's lace. Dr. Kurt Schaunbelt considers carrot seed oil as one of the strongest revitalizing essential oils.

- Known for its care of dry or damaged skin and hair, dermatitis, eczema and rashes
- Restores elasticity and helps to eliminate wrinkles

- Helps to encourage the growth of new skin cells and improve skin tone
- May slow progression of wrinkles, increases blood circulation, improves liver function
- May be added to face creams for general skin health
- High in vitamin A and beta carotene
- High amounts in antioxidant vitamins C and E—help to counteract free radical damage.

It leads the way in plant extracts that deliver Vitamin A which is excellent for skin repair and collagen production.

Cedarwood (Cedrus atlantica)
Code: D, O, N

- May be beneficial for skin disorders such as acne, rashes and psoriasis.
- It is beneficial to the skin and tissues near the surface of the skin.
- It is high in sesquiterpenes that can stimulate the limbic region of the brain (the center of the emotions).
- It may also help stimulate the pineal gland to release melatonin, an antioxidant hormone associated with deep sleep and anti-aging.
- Controls dandruff, improves circulation and condition of the hair, stimulates hair follicles; reduces cellulite.

Chamomile (Chamaemelum nobile)
Code: D, M, N, O

Is a powerful relaxant and anti-inflammatory. Used in Europe to decongest with facial steam.

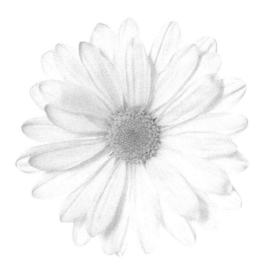

- Calming to irritated skin, relieves discomforts of psoriasis, eczema, dermatis and sunburn
- Reduces dryness, itching, redness, and sensitivity in irritated and inflamed skin
- Soothes dry, sensitive skin
- Can reduce redness of fragile capillaries
- Condition hair, scalp; adds shine and lustre

Clary Sage (Salvia sclarea)
Code: D, O, W, M

- Clary Sage is anti-infectious, (thus excellent for poor skin conditions) exhibits moderate antibacterial activity against various strains of bacteria:
- Listeria monocytogenes, Staphylococcus aureus, Klebsiella & has potent anti-fungal activity against strains of Candida, Aspergillus & Penicillium.

- Eases menopausal discomfort, menstrual pain, PMS/ regulates menstrual cycles. Due to its esters, Is anti-spasmodic (relaxes muscular spasms/pains), relaxes the nerves from stress and nervous tension
- Has strong estrogen-like properties (hence not to be used during pregnancy) Supports hormones, regulates blood pressure
- Helps treat symptoms of chronic fatigue syndrome
- Supports healthy digestion
- Improves memory/ stimulates mental activity
- Helps for various respiratory ailments including asthma, bronchitis, sore throat, colds.
- Clary Sage Essential Oil is high in Antioxidants and provides outstanding benefits for your eyes, nervous system, digestion, skin and kidneys.
- Clary sage's name originates from the Latin word "clarus," which means "clear."
- During the Middle Ages it was referred to as "clear eyes".
- Clary essential oil is added to soaps, detergents, creams, lotions, and perfumes. Interestingly, it is the main component of
- Eau de Cologne.

**Use this oil with caution if there is an estrogen-induced condition due to its estrogenic nature, clary sage essential oil may have a negative impact on people. Seek the advice of a healthcare professional

- Apply topically as a moisturizer to regulate the production of sebum on your skin.
- Regulates oil production and reduces inflammation that contributes to dermatitis.
- Promotes regeneration of skin cells
- Improves acne, seborrhea, dry skin
- Helps with hair growth
- Helps ward off wrinkles, keeps skin looking healthy and youthful

Copaiba (Copaifera reticulata/langsdorfii)
Code: D, O, W, M
- Used extensively in spiritual practices, emotional first aid, equalizer
- Helps to reduce stress and balance emotions
- Traditional uses in Amazon has been for stomach ulcers and cancer
- Due to its anti-inflammatory properties , it is excellent for sore muscles/ back pain/carpal tunnel syndrome and urinary problems, bronchitis and tuberculosis

- The oil is usually applied to the skin to soften it. It has a naturally high content of essential fatty acids which are the building blocks for the skin's tissues.
- Copaiba oleoresin appears to have an anti-cancer action on metastatic lung tumour cells and also on melanoma (skin cancer) cells
- Acne – Because of its super anti-inflammatory power, it reduces redness around the acne rather quickly. Apply 2 drops of this oil on a cotton ball and dab it directly (without diluting) on active area. Use daily.
- Stretch Marks – Apply the oil directly on stretch marks to fade them. Use this in conjugation with olive oil to fade stretch marks.
- Sagging Skin – Apply it direct on skin areas which are sagging. Copaiba oil boosts secretion of collagen and elastin to make skin firm and taut.
- Skin disorders – Apply the oil directly over the area: Helps skin such as psoriasis, eczema and dermatitis
- Insect bites – Apply the oil directly over the inflamed bite.

Cypress (Cupressus sempervirens)
Code: O
May be beneficial for arthritis, circulation, cramps, insomnia, menopausal problems, menstrual pain, varicose veins, and fluid retention.

- Beneficial for oily skin, hair, acne and dandruff
- Deodorizing and controls excessive bodily secretions, thus great to use as a deodorant
- Stops bleeding of nick and cuts
- Constricts blood vessels beneficial – for broken capillaries and varicose veins
- Diminish or prevent stretch marks
- Great for cellulite as it strengthens weak connective tissues, improves circulation and helps release toxin

Elemi (Canarium luzonicum)
Code: D, O, N, W
Has cell-regeneration properties/same botanical family as Frankincense

- Rejuvenating for wrinkled, sagging skin
- Balances sebum secretions
- Controls heavy perspiration
- Used in Europe in salves for the skin

Frankincense (Boswelia carteri)
Code: D, O, N, W
It has been known for centuries for its beautifying properties. The ancient Egyptians used it in rejuvenation face masks.

- The restorative, regenerating and rejuvenating actions are especially useful for dry, mature/sensitive skin.
- Smoothes lines and wrinkles. Frankincense has properties that renew cells to their original state, thus promoting younger looking skin. It will reduce the appearance of wrinkles and prevent new wrinkles from forming.
- Soothes and softens raw skin
- Balances oily skin
- Accelerates the healing of blemishes, inflammations, sores, scars, skin ulcers and wounds
- Dry Skin Treatment – Frankincense oil works as a super-nourishing dry skin treatment, especially for mature and aging skin.

Geranium (Pelargonium graveolens)
Code: D, O, N, W
Has been used for centuries in skin care.

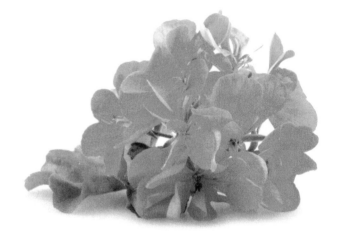

- Excellent for skin
- Helpful to any skin type; revitalizes skin tissue and treats a long list of skin problems
- Regenerate skin cells and speeds healing of acne and blemishes
- Soothes dry, sensitive skin
- Imparts a healthy glow, giving skin a radiant and youthful appearance
- Stimulates both lymphatic and
- circulatory systems – helpful for cellulite
- Balances sebum (fatty secretion in the sebaceous glands of the skin that keep the skin supple)
- Helps smooth lines and wrinkles, and is said to slow the skin's aging process

Helichrysum (Helichrysum italicum)
Code: M, O
Also known as immortelle or everlasting, appropriately named for its anti-aging properties

The health benefits of Helichrysum Essential Oil can be attributed to its many healing & health properties as an antispasmodic, anticoagulant, antiallergenic, antimicrobial, anti-haematoma, antiphlogistic, nervine, diuretic, hepatic, fungicidal, anti-inflammatory, and many other attributes. Helichrysum oil is known for its restorative properties and provides excellent support to the skin, liver, and nervous system. Use for combating minor aches and pains associated with everyday life or exercise.

Other attributes:

- Antibacterial, anti-fungal, mucolytic
- Antioxidant
- Anti-catarrhal

Stimulates new cell formation.

- Indicated for healing bruises, open wounds and cuts, varicose veins, acne, eczema and psoriasis.
- Supports and regenerates tissue and nerves, healthy skin and circulation
- Improves itching, redness, scaliness of psoriasis, eczema, acne
- Restorative properties to mature skin
- Effective sunscreen
- Scores high – 17,430 on the antioxidant ORAC scale

Jasmine (Jasminum officinale)
Code: D, O, N, M (an absolute)

- Benefits any skin type, including sensitive skin (hot, inflamed skin)
- Inhibits bacteria, regulates oil production, helps with acne and oily skin
- Helps moisturize dry, dehydrated or mature skin
- Anti-depressant
- Very uplifting, increases self confidence, relaxing, relieves stress
- Hormonal regulator

Juniper Berry (Juniperus osteoperma)
Code: O

Juniper increases circulation through kidneys and promotes excretion of uric acid and toxins. It may help acne, dermatitis, eczema, depression, fatigue, sore muscles, fluid retention and wounds.

- Nerve regeneration, beneficial for the skin
- Promotes cellular wastes and stimulates circulation
- Enlivens dull skin, regulated oily skin
- Good for varicose veins and cellulite

Lavender (Lavanduala angustifolia)
Code: D, N, M (Good for all skin types.)

- Powerful relaxant and a strong yet gentle antiseptic.
- Calms and soothes the skin,
- stimulates circulation.
- May be used for burns (cell renewal), sunburns (including lips),
- dandruff,

- hair loss
- allergies,
- headaches,
- insomnia,
- menopause,
- PMS, scarring, acne, dermatitis, eczema, psoriasis and rashes. and dark spots

Lemon (Citrus limona) *
Code: O, D, W

- Is an astringent skin toner; has a mild bleaching action
- Helps to clear acne, minimizes corns and warts
- Brightens a pale, dull complexion by removing dead skin cells
- Reduces cellulite, broken capillaries and varicose veins, excellent for lymphatic stasis
- Helps to reduce puffiness and wrinkles
- Strengthens fingernails

*Do Not use before going out into the sun

Lemongrass (Cymbopogon flexuosus)
Code: O, N

Supports digestion, tones and helps regenerate connective tissues and ligaments, dilates blood vessels, known as a headache remedy, strengthens vascular walls, promotes lymph flow, is anti-inflammatory, a sedative and reduces swelling.

- Also good for sagging, devitalized smoker's skin – helps to eliminate wastes
- Scores 17,765 on the antioxidant ORAC scale
- Effective cleanser for oily skin with acne

Melaleuca (Tea Tree) (Melaleuca alternifolia)
Code: O, N

- Rivals benzoyl peroxide for effectiveness in fighting acne and no side effects
- Great for aftershave irritation and infection of ingrown hairs
- Fungal infection, sunburn
- Hastens the healing of wounds, diaper rash, acne and insect bites
- Protects skin from radiation burns, encourages the regeneration of scar tissue and reduces swelling
- Oil controlling agent

Myrrh (Commiphora myrrha)
Code: D, W, M

Essential Desk Reference – "The Arabian people used Myrrh for many skin conditions, such as chapped and cracked skin and wrinkles."

- Maintains healthy skin
- Prevents premature aging of the skin
- Soothes and softens dried, chapped lips
- Claims made that it wards off wrinkles (a prized ingredient for stretch marks and wrinkles)
- Regenerates skin cells, reduces inflammation, fights infection, heals wounds
- Improves circulation – helps skin look smoother and more youthful
- Heals blemishes, skin ulcers and wounds, ringworm, eczema and psoriasis

Orange (Citrus sinensis)
Code: O, W, M

Helps complexion (dull and oily), dermatitis, mouth ulcers, muscle soreness, sedation, tissue repair, fluid retention and wrinkles.

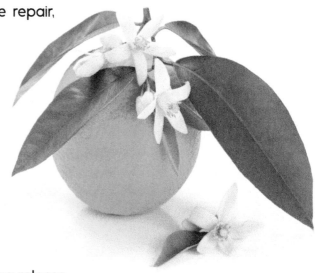

- Maintains healthy skin
- Promotes production of collagen
- Reduces puffiness
- Discourages dry or wrinkled skin
- Softens rough skin
- Clears blemishes and improves acne-prone skin
- Increases perspiration, assisting release of toxins.
- Improves cellulite

*Do Not use before going out into the sun

** Orchid Oil – See below

Palmarosa (Cymbopogon martini)
Code: O, N, M
- antibacterial, antifungal, antiviral, supports heart and nervous system
- Essential Oil of Palma Rosa curbs and inhibits the duplication of the virus and successfully eliminates it.

- stimulates new skin cell growth
- regulates sebum production in skin
- good for skin problems- acne, eczema
- fungal infections/candida
- It keeps the skin soft, moist, and looking young.
- Helps cure sores, cracks on the skin and Athlete's Foot.
- Aids digestion

Patchouly (Pogostemon cablin)
Code: D, O, N, W

Beneficial for the skin and may help prevent wrinkles or chapped skin. It is also anti- micro-bial, antiseptic, and helps relieve itching, allergies, dermatitis, eczema, hemorrhoids and regenerates tissue.

- Tightens and tones sagging skin
- Speeds healing of sores and wounds, fades scars
- Soothes inflamed skin
- Repels insects
- Reduces fluid retention and tightens saggy skin; beneficial for cellulite
  — Acts as a deodorant

Pine Oil (Pinus sylvestris)
Code: D, O, M

- hormone-like, cortisone-like, antiseptic, lymphatic stimulant
- good for skin parasites
- relieves anxiety and revitalizes mind, body and spirit.
- disinfectant
- has the ability to reduce inflammation and associated redness,
- aid the body in cleansing impurities,
- fight off sinus infections,
- clear mucus and phlegm,
- cure skin conditions like eczema and psoriasis*,
- boost your immune system,
- fight fungal and viral infections (great for colds and flus),
- relieve anxiety (anxio-lytic effect)

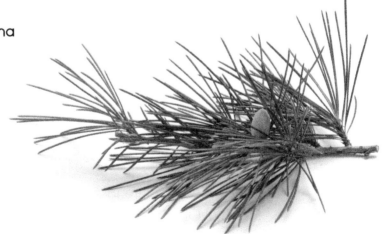

*Dermatologists often prescribe this oil for treating psoriasis, itching, pimples, eczema, skin diseases, poor skin, scabies, sores, and fleas. Frequent use helps to keep the skin smooth, renewed and shiny and also acts as an antioxidant for free radicals.

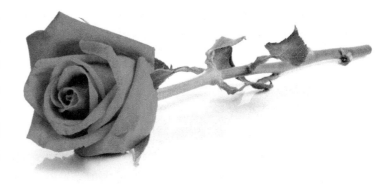

Word of Caution: Avoid any pine essential oils adulterated with turpentine, low-cost, but potentially hazardous filler. Hence the reason it is most important to know your company

Rose Oil (Rosa damascena)
Code: D, N, W, M

Cleopatra's cosmetics contained actual roses. Rose oil has been used for the skin for thousands of years to help skin cells absorb and retain moisture, leaving the surface hydrated, healthy and smooth.

- Helps to restore the moisture balance and smoothes wrinkles
- Helps to diminish the redness of broken capillaries;
- Anti-inflammatory
- Benefits all skin types; dry, sensitive, and mature skin.
- Rose is an excellent treatment for inflamed skin, allergies, psoriasis, atopic dermatitis and eczema
- Cell rejuvenator
- Reduces scarring
- Has been shown to have a positive effect in treating depression.
- Rose oil can also help refine skin texture.
- Rose essential oil can help heal wounds, it inhibits water loss in the skin and inhaling it lowers the concentration of cortisol (a stress hormone) in the body.
- Improves memory/ stimulates mental activity
- Helps for various respiratory ailments including asthma, bronchitis, sore throat, colds.

-

Rose is among the most treasured essential oils due to its holistic ability to gently soothe and clear the skin. Use as a skin-quenching facial toner or mist — by adding a few drops to your 8 oz spray bottle, Shake and spritz.

Rosehip Seed Oil (Rosa rubiginosa)
Code: N, W

- For wrinkles. Found to be effective in tissue regeneration.
- Healing effect on chronic ulcerations of the skin, skin grafts, brown spots and prematurely aging skin, and prevents skin dehydration.
- Excellent oil to use on the skin after sun treatment.
- Has wonderful skin rejuvenating properties.
- This oil is used directly on the skin;
- Fights photo aging, reduces surgical and trauma scars.
- Contains unique plant compounds that are included in some of the most powerful skin treatments. The best quality of rosehip seed oil is currently produced in Chile where it was clinically tested at the University of Santiago. Creer Laboratory provides the same organic clinically tested oil.
  - (See resources)

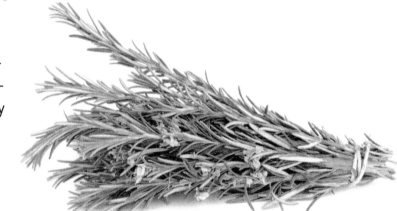

- Rich in vitamin C, A, B, E and K; contains essential fatty acids and tretinoin – the most beneficial property of rosehip seed oil.
- It is the only vegetable oil that naturally contains retinol (vitamin A), which may helps to treat lines and wrinkles and other visible signs of aging.
- Rosehip oil has been shown to inhibit pigmentation, which often shows up as "age spots"
- or sun spots, so may be found in sunscreens, skin lighteners, and other anti-aging crèmes.
- Rosewater is soothing and nourishing. Use as a facial mist.

Rosemary Verbenon (Rosmarinus officinalis)
Code: D, O, W, N

Known for stimulating new cell formation. Can benefit all skin types and particularly good in regenerating, nurturing the skin.

- Eases lines and wrinkles
- Nourishes the scalp
- Heals wounds
- Improves circulation
- Clears acne

Rosewood (Aniba rosaeodora)
Code: D, O, N, W

- Stimulates new cell growth
- Regenerates tissue, soothing to the skin
- Minimizes lines and wrinkles
- Balances dry or oily skin
- Clear blemishes, improves acne
- May create skin elasticity

Sage (Salvia officinalis)
Code: O, N

- Astringent properties – ideal for oily skin and hair
- Effective for dandruff
- Stimulating to the lymphatic system and glandular system
- Regulates hormonal function (hot flushes/menstrual period)
- Tonifying to the circulatory system and nervous system (exhaustion)
- Soothes skin conditions, reduces scarring

Sandalwood (Santalum album)
Code: D, O, N, W, M

Sandalwood is high in sesquiterpenes that have been researched in Europe for their ability to stimulate the pineal gland and the limbic region of the brain, the center of emotions. The pineal gland is responsible for releasing melatonin, a powerful antioxidant that enhances deep sleep and supports nerves and circulation.

- Relieves itching and irritation after shaving
- Nourishes dry, dehydrated and mature skin
- Smooths and softens lines and wrinkles
- Good for any skin type; clears acne
- Makes an effective deodorant

Spikenard (Nardostachys jatamansi)
Code: D, N, M

- Regenerates the skin
- Good for skin tone, rashes, allergies, skin eruptions
- Bacterial infections
- Wounds that will not heal

Sulfur

Keeps the skin smooth and youthful. Best taken internally and can be used externally as well. Best source is methysulfonylmethane (MSM). It is found in garlic, onions, eggs, asparagus and amino acid L-cysteine. YL product: Sulferzyme.

Twelve Oils of Ancient Scripture
Code: D, M, O, N
A special spiritual kit containing 12 oils mentioned in Scriptures: Aloes/Sandalwood, Cassia,

Cedarwood, Cypress, Galbanum, Frankincense, Hyssop, Myrrh, Calamus, Myrtle, Onycha,

Rose of Sharon. Any or all of these oils can be used for the face.

Vetiver (Vetiveria zizaniodies)
- Improves circulation and immunity
- Clears acne, replenishes moisture in dry and dehydrated skin
- Strengthens connective tissue
- Rejuvenating effect on the complexion (mature skin)
- Prized in skin care for its deep penetration, plumping up thin and sagging skin tissues
- Heals cuts and wounds
- Soothes irritated and inflamed skin
- Use as a deodorizer

Ylang Ylang (Cananga odorata)
Code: D, N, O, W
- Benefits any skin type, especially helpful for oily skin
- Controls acne and blemishes
- Softens and smooths skin, and stimulates new cell growth
- Can ward off wrinkles and premature aging as it relaxes facial muscles and releases facial tension

Orchid Flower Oil: A Special Feature
Ancient tradition has revered the orchid flower as a symbol of perfection and beauty for thousands of years—It was known to nourish, hydrate and restore vitality to the skin.

Young Living is the only company that has combined the antiaging benefits of the orchid oil powers with pure essential oils.

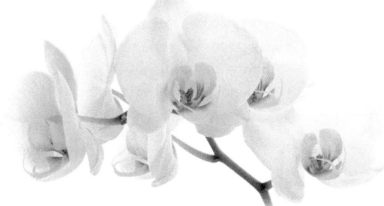

- The orchid symbolizes virtue in Chinese tradition.
- It is a symbol of nobility, friendship and love.
- Orchid petals contain many moisturizing ingredients and are highly valued for their reparative and protective properties.
- Orchid oil has the ability to fight free radicals and protect the skin from effects of pollution
- Dermatologists have considered the orchid as a "perfect plant" for the skin;
- as the orchid moisturizes,
- boosts skin immunity,
- reduces fine lines, and soothes.
- It also has skin-fortifying minerals like calcium, magnesium, and zinc. And it's an antioxidant to boot.
- Orchid oil seems to Firm, Tone, Clarify, Lighten, Reduce lines, forehead folds and gives the skin that elusive glow!
- The Serum and the masque are superb in their ability to help restore elasticity.

THE MANY VIRTUES OF ESSENTIAL OILS

AROMAS

Spirit

- Awakens the spirit

Mind

- Quiets the mind
- Reduces stress and anxiety
- Soothes emotions

Skin

- Rejuvenates the skin (increases circulation)
- Renews the cells
- Revitalizes the skin
- Rehydrates and repairs collagen
- Reverses aging of the skin
- Reduces puffiness and inflammation, and wrinkles

Body

- Normalizes heart rate
- Restores homeostasis
- Balances hormones
- Relaxes muscles
- Boosts immunity

SPECIAL TIPS FOR ACNE

Acne can be a major problem for teenagers, but can appear at any age. Acne is often the result of the oil- producing glands, sebaceous glands, over producing sebum or oil. As a result, an overgrowth of bacteria together with the blocked sebum causes pimples to form. As mentioned earlier, a holistic approach is recommended to treat this common skin problem.

A hormonal imbalance, along with a toxic condition of the liver, kidneys and intestines is often blamed as the cause of acne. Toxic foods, sugar, fatty foods, toxic cosmetic ingredients as presented earlier in this book—i.e., fragrances, preservatives, pesticides, environmental pollution, oral contraceptive, stress, emotional problems and sunscreens all contribute to this skin problem.

1. Start an intense cleansing (colon and liver) program—use products like Cleansing Trio from Young Living or others readily available from health food stores. Parasites, Candida, bacterial infestation is critical to cleanse. Cleansing Trio contains Juva Tone a liver cleansing tablet and ICP, a high fiber bowel powder to help cleanse the liver and bowels.

   ADD good **quality Probiotics** to your daily regimen so as to rebalance the pH and intestinal flora.

   Cleanse face with Melaleuca-Geranium bar soap or Lemon-Sandalwood bar soap. Or make your own cleanser—Use R. Wilson's Clay Cleanser below.

   Mix into a paste:

   - 1 tsp. clay powder
   - 1 tsp. honey (or water)
   - 1 drop Geranium oil
   - 1 drop Lavender oil
   - 1 drop Melaleuca oil

2. Avoid fried foods, sugar, dairy and chemical products. Stimulants of any kind need to be avoided.

   Alcohol, coffee, tea, chocolate and smoking aggravate the condition. Caffeine and sugar combined in chocolate make it doubly worse for acne. It is preferable to eat lots of green vegetables, not fruit (due to its high sugar content, fruit can make acne worse).

   Antibiotics are often prescribed for this skin condition which only treats the symptoms temporarily and wipes out friendly intestinal bacteria. This only makes the matter worse and creates a situation for Candida – yeast overgrowth to thrive.

3. Avoid cosmetics containing colors, dyes, fragrances and preservatives.

4. Topically apply **Melaleuca Alternifolia** (as effective as most common over-the-counter acne medication—benzoyl peroxide) or **Eucalyptus Dives** or any of these combinations:

   - Use **carrot oil** instead of Retin A (contains natural vitamin A and extremely rich in beta carotene)
   - **Frankincense** and **Melaleuca Alternifolia**
   - **Melaleuca** with **Lemon, Lemongrass, Thyme, Basil** or **Geranium**
   - **Melrose** and **Gentle Baby**
   - **Vetiver oil, Sandalwood, Copaiba**
   - Combine 1/2 oz. jojoba oil, 8 drops **Lavender**, 4 drops **Melaleuca**, 3 drops Cypress and 2 drops **Helichrysum**. Dab blemish several times daily.
   - Create your own acne paste. K. Keville recommends combine 12 drops Tea Tree oil into 1/2 teaspoon comfrey root powder with 1 tablespoon distilled water. Mix well and dab on acne spots. Let dry for 20 minutes or so. Rinse off.
   - Apply Clary Sage by dabbing on the spots

5. Eat wholesome nutritious foods—remember lots of green vegetables. Get daily fresh air and exercise. Breathe deeply.

6. Follow the weekly regime of scrub, steaming your face and face mask. Proper skin care is crucial for clearing this problem. Cleanse 2 times a day. Spot treat blemishes with essential oils throughout the day.

7. Use Rosemary CT cineol or Eucalyptus Dives essential oils for your steam bath

8. Include Evening Primrose Oil capsules to help prevent recurring acne.

9. Most importantly- get your hormones and Endocrine glands checked and balanced by using a natural approach.

10. Supplement daily 10,000 IU beta carotene, 1000–2000 mg vitamin C, 20–25 mg zinc. Drink fresh carrot juice, beet juice and detoxifying herbal teas.

Add supplements to balance your thyroid, adrenals or other endocrine imbalances.

ESSENTIAL OIL GUIDELINES

ANTI-INFLAMMATORY OILS (REDUCE SWELLING)	BALANCING OILS (NORMALIZE OILINESS)	ASTRINGENT OILS (CONTROL OILINESS)
Blue Cyprus	Clary Sage	Cedarwood
Chamomile	Bergamot	Cypress
Clary Sage	Cypress	Clary Sage
Frankincense	Elemi	Geranium
Geranium	Geranium	Frankincense
Helichrysum	Lavender	Orange
Patchouli	Lemon	Patchouli
Oregano	Orange	Rosewood
Rosewood	Rose	Ylang Ylang
Lavender	Sandalwood	
Nutmeg	Ylang Ylang	
Peppermint		

A NOTE ABOUT THE SUN

Since intense sun exposure is the most damaging to the skin, it is the most important to take precautionary measures.

- Minimize exposure to the sun, especially between 11:00 a.m. and 3:00 p.m.
- Wear hats and clothing that cover much of your body.
- Wear sunglasses to filter out harmful UV rays.
- Always use a natural sunscreen. Unfortunately, most opt for the many commercial sunscreens that contain harsh chemicals, which actually encourage the formation of cancer cells on the skin. Many dermatologists discourage the use for moderate to dark- colored skin.

Certain natural vegetable oils and essential oils have been found to provide some protection against the sun. I often ask, what did the Egyptians use? They certainly didn't use toxic chemicals but all natural unguents and ointments made with oils, waxes and essential oils.

Sesame oil can block or reduce about 30% of the burning rays; coconut and olive oils about 20% and aloe vera inhibits about 20%. Sea Buckthorn oil can also be used to **Prevent A Sunburn** when mixed with lavender or helichrysum oil. **Helichrysum oil** has been researched for its ability to effectively screen out some of the sun's rays. Listed below are some essential oil blends.

Sunblock

Mix 3–6 drops **Helichrysum** (Helichrysum italicum) with 100 drops of sesame oil or olive oil. Apply on skin every few hours.

According to R. Wilson, as suggested in her book **Aromatherapy**, the following blend below will serve as a reliable sunscreen.

Natural Sunscreen

- 1 oz. sesame oil
- 1/2 oz. olive oil
- 5 drops Lavender

- 1/2 oz. coconut oil
- 10 drops Helichrysum
- 3 drops Chamomile

Mix and apply.

For Sunburn Relief—(if this should happen to you)

1. **LavaDerm Cooling Mist** by Young Living contains Lavender and aloe vera, both known to alleviate burns effectively and immediately. Spray burn immediately with the mist and often (every 10 minutes) followed by 2–3 drops of **Lavender Oil**.

2. Apply any of these oils to relieve discomfort/inflammation: **Chamomile, Helichrysum, Peppermint** (mix 1 drop with a carrier or mixing oil, then apply)

3. Blend and apply:
   - 2 oz. sesame oil
   - 5 drops Helichrysum
   - 2 drops Patchouli or 5 drops Geranium

   - 12–25 drops Lavender
   - 4 drops Chamomile

4. Apply Mineral Essence (a liquid trace mineral supplement by Young Living) to the burn. Or purchase a liquid mineral from the health store. Add to a spray bottle with a few drops of lavender oil and spray the painful area.

According to Dr. Alex Schauss, a prominent researcher, educator, burns are painful because the skin is lacking certain trace minerals. When replenished, the pain will subside.

CHAPTER 11

ESSENTIAL OIL FORMULAS

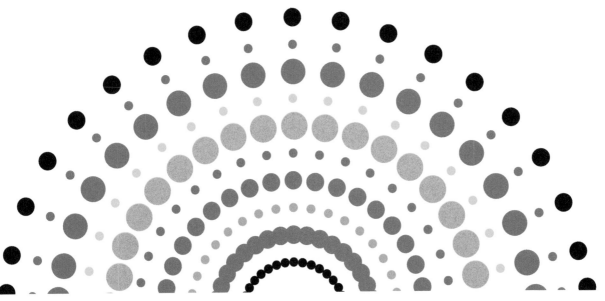

*"It may take you a little longer to reach peak potential
when you are ninety but, even at that age,
the essential oils can make you feel and look younger."*
VALARIE ANN WORWOOD

ESSENTIAL OILS FOR SAGGING SKIN

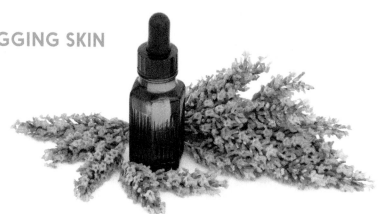

- Blue Cypress
- Lavender
- Copaiba
- Patchouli
- Helichrysum
- Cypress
- Lemongrass

Add any of the above oils to Cel-Lite Magic, a carrier oil mix by Young Living or any carrier oil of your choice & Massage on location.

MORNING ROUTINE*

- 10 drops Tangerine
- 10 drops Cypress
- Mix with oil base and massage.

SPECIAL NECK TREATMENT (V.A. WORWOOD) BLEND

Blend together:
- 10 drops Rose
- 7 drops Clary Sage
- 10 drops Lemon
- 20 drops Carrot Seed Oil

Add in one teaspoon evening primrose oil. Massage well into the neck. Leave on for 10 minutes, then wipe off excess.

EVENING ROUTINE *

- 8 drops Geranium
- 5 drops Cypress
- 5 drops Helichrysum
- 1 drop Peppermint

Mix with oil base. Apply to location, seal with Cel-Lite Magic, product by Young Living Company.

SPECIAL TONER FOR SAGGING SKIN

- 1 drop Neroli
- 1 drop Helichrysum

Combine 1 oz. evening primrose oil or borage oil. Apply to cotton pad and wipe face after cleansing.

(*Above recipes excerpted from PDR, Essential Science Publishing)

ESSENTIAL OILS FOR WRINKLES

- Rosewood
- Rose Oil
- Rosehip Seed Oil
- Frankincense
- Cypress
- Geranium
- Lavender
- Patchouli
- Ylang Ylang
- Sandalwood
- Myrrh
- Lemon
- Clary Sage
- Orange
- Blue Cypress
- Rosemary
- Thyme
- Helichrysum
- Carrot

Keep the mind young and alert: Bergamot is stimulating, uplifting, go-getting, calming, relaxes brain waves and can be used as an anti-depressant. Also serves as an effective deodorant (kills odor-causing bacteria)!

BELOW ARE PROPRIETARY BLENDS BY YOUNG LIVING COMPANY THAT ARE WONDERFUL FOR SKIN CARE:

Sensation Oil Blend™ Proprietary Blend

(Contains: Coriandrum Sativum (**Coriander**) seed oil, Cananga odorata (**Ylang ylang**) flower oil, Citrus aurantium bergamia (Furanocoumarin-free **Bergamot**) peel oil, Jasminum officinale (**Jasmine**) oil, Pelargonium graveolens (**Geranium**) flower oil.

- Very uplifting and refreshing
- Very nourishing and hydrating for the skin
- Beneficial for various skin problems
- Exotic and extremely uplifting and refreshing.
- It can also enhance the enjoyment of special moments.

Add 1–2 drops of this blend to your moisturizing formulas and can add to your masks.

BUILD YOUR DREAM™ PROPRIETARY BLEND

Lavender (Lavandula angustifolia†), Sacred Frankincense (Boswellia sacra†), melissa (Melissa officinalis†), blue cypress (Callitris intratropica†), hong kuai (Chamaecyparis formosensis†), Idaho blue spruce (Picea pungens†), ylang ylang (Cananga odorata†), Dream Catcher™ (Sandalwood, Black Pepper, Anise, Tangerine, Bergamot, Blue Tansy, Ylang Ylang, Juniper), Believe (Idaho Blue Spruce, Idaho Balsam Fir, Frankincense, Coriander, Bergamot, Ylang Ylang, Geranium), blue lotus (Nymphaea caerulea†)

In 2014 Young Living Company marked their two decades for setting the high standard for quality, purity and effectiveness in the essential oils industry. CEO and founder D. Gary Young formulated this unique, commemorative blend, called "**Build Your Dream.**"

This powerful blend offers many benefits: inspires calmness, uplifts emotions, boosts spiritual awareness and enlightenment, increases feelings of self-confidence, and promotes desire to expand potential.

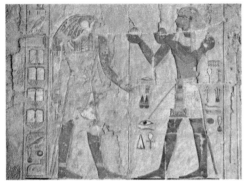

The essential oils contained in this blend are also helpful for skin care, by supporting healthy-looking, vibrant skin, especially with the addition of the rare and exotic **Blue Lotus oil.

*ABOUT BLUE LOTUS:

*Only the kings, according to ancient legend, had access to the blue lotus oil which gave them great spiritual powers as well as protecting them from death. It was said that those who "possessed the **Blue Lotus** would never have sickness" (Young, pg.12, 1996).

Gary Young in his book *"Aromatherapy, The Essential Beginning"* points out how the Blue Lotus was also used in religious rituals as offerings to their gods giving them great favor and putting them in good standing. It was also used to heal tumors, blindness, baldness, stomach sicknesses—and liver formulations included lotus leaves in their concoctions.

Add 1–2 drops of this blend to your moisturizing formulas and this blend can also be added to your masks. Enjoy a most exquisite experience.

GENTLE BABY BLEND™ PROPRIETARY BLEND

(Contains: **Palmarosa, Geranium, Roman Chamomile, Rose, Lavender, Rosewood, Ylang Ylang, Bergamot, Jasmine and Lemon**)

- Improves skin elasticity
- Smoothes wrinkles
- Reduces stretch marks and scar tissue
- Enhances youthful appearance

Add 1–2 drops of this blend to your moisturizing formulas and can add to your masks.

STRESS AWAY BLEND™ PROPRIETARY BLEND

Stress Away™ contains: **Copaiba** (Copaifera reticulata), **Lime** (Citrus aurantifolia), **Cedarwood** (Cedrus atlantica), **Vanilla** (Vanilla planifolia), **Ocotea** (Ocotea quixos), **Lavender** (Lavandula angustifolia)

Stress Away is the perfect on-the-go natural solution to combat normal stresses that creep into our everyday lives. It is the first product to contain the unique stress-relieving combination of lime and vanilla pure, therapeutic-grade essential oils. Both the copaiba and lavender oils help to reduce mental rigidity and restore equilibrium. Other powerful plant constituents, such as the cedrol found in cedarwood and the eugenol that occurs naturally in vanilla, help to make Stress Away a unique blend in inducing relaxation and reducing occasional nervous tension.*

The unique blend of **Vanilla**, with its warm, sweet aroma, calms and reduces tension. (Also see more on Vanilla for facial masks in chapter 12).

LIME – the delicious scent of lime is robust and refreshing.

OCOTEA – has a cinnamon base with a kick of exotic luxury.

CEDARWOOD – with one of the highest known levels of sesquiterpenes, works with the brain to improve relaxation.

COPAIBA – supports the Stress Away blend with the powerful constituents' beta caryo-phyllene an anti-inflammatory property which makes it excellent for sore muscles/back pain/ and many other inflammatory issues.

LAVENDER – the floral scent of lavender is calming and eases tension.

Benefits: Reduce stress anytime, anywhere with the Use of Stress Away. Helps to relax facial muscles if used in your facial routine and reduce mental tension via inhalation.

Lessening normal everyday stress can lead to improved sleep, telomere enhancement, reduction in cortisol preventing adrenal burn-out and elevated state of mind.

Add 1–2 drops of this blend to your moisturizing formulas and can add to your masks.

OTHER OILS FOR MOISTURIZING EFFECTS:

- Frankincense
- Myrrh
- Clary Sage
- Rose
- Jasmine
- Lavender
- Patchouli
- Sandalwood

You can add any of the above oils to any of your favourite creams or carrier oil. Here are a few suggestions that are from Young Living Company below:

- Boswellia Wrinkle Créme
- Sheer-Lume™ (a new YL crème)
- Sandalwood Moisture Créme
- Wolfberry Eye Créme

Choose your Carrier oil from the list below that best suits your needs. Three or four of these carrier oils can be combined as well along with the essential oils in an 8 oz. bottle. Create your own that is best suited for your skin type and lifestyle needs.

MORE SAGGING SKIN TIPS

1. **Egg White**

    Egg whites are popularly used as a natural astringent and hence work as a good remedy for sagging skin. Its skin-nourishing ingredient of emollients and emulsifiers help to lubricate the skin and lift loose skin.

    *   Simple to use—Whisk one to two egg whites until you get a foamy texture. Add 1 drop cypress or lavender. Apply it to the face and neck. Leave it on for about 20 minutes and then rinse it off with cool water.
    *   Another option is to add one tablespoon of plain yogurt to one egg white and whisk it. Add

        —   1 drop cypress, lavender, patchouli or lemongrass. Apply the mixture to your face and neck and leave it on for 20 to 30 minutes before rinsing it off. You can use either of these remedies twice a week to enjoy firm, radiant, glowing skin.

2. **Lemon**

    Due to lemon's vitamin C content, it helps to boost collagen production which in turn helps restore elasticity to your skin. Lemon also has astringent properties that help tighten the skin and reduce wrinkles and other signs of premature aging.

    *   Extract some fresh lemon juice Add 1–2 drops of lemon essential oil to it. Rub it gently on your face and neck. Leave it on for five to 10 minutes and then rinse your face with water. Do this two times a day followed with a good-quality moisturizer.
    *   You can also add the juice of half a lemon with the lemon oil to a cup of cold water. Splash this mixture on your freshly washed face. Let the lemon water air dry on your face. Do this once or twice daily for best results.

3. **Power of Aloe**

The Egyptians called Aloe Vera the "Plant of Immortality" and beauties like Nefertiti and Cleopatra depended on aloe vera for smooth skin.

Alexander the Great and Christopher Columbus always had aloe handy.

Fresh Aloe Vera gel is best to use for this procedure. Aloe Vera firms and tightens loose skin. The malic acid in aloe vera gel helps improve the elasticity of your skin as well as lift sagging skin. Plus, it is a natural moisturizer for your skin.

Simple steps to Use the Aloe Vera gel from your plant

1. Cut an aloe leaf from your plant using a sharp knife. Cut off about two inches from the base of the plant — store the remaining aloe vera leaf upright in a jar. Rinse the leaf to cleanse it.

2. Cut off the green skin on the flat side of the leaf and scoop out the gel inside with a spoon.

3. Use on its own to smear on your face and neck or add 1 drop of Frankincense or Helichrysum essential oil. Leave it on for 15 to 20 minutes and then wash it off with lukewarm water. Can also leave it on overnight and wash in the morning. Follow this remedy several times a week for an aloe vera facial!

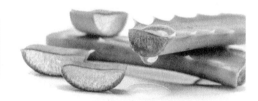

4. **Honey**

Honey has been widely used and known for its natural hydrating, antioxidant and anti aging properties that are helpful for treating sagging skin. Honey works well with other mixtures and essential oils.

- Mix two to three teaspoons of honey with a few drops each of lemon juice and olive oil. Apply it on your face and neck, let it dry and then rinse it off with warm water. Do this once or twice daily for best results.
- Another variation, Mix together one-half tablespoon each of honey and sour cream. Then mix in one-half teaspoon of turmeric powder. Add 2 drops of helichrysum or lavender oil. Apply to your face and leave it for 15 minutes. Rinse it off with lukewarm water and then splash some cold water. Use this face mask once a week.

5. Strawberry

Strawberries work very well as an astringent on the skin, making them a natural home remedy for sagging skin. Make sure that they are organic.

Strawberries are high in vitamin C, a potent antioxidant that boosts production of collagen fibers that help to smooth and firm the skin. They also contain the alpha hydroxyl acids that help to improve the appearance of aging skin.

- Mash two to three ripe strawberries and mix them with two teaspoons each of yogurt and honey. Add Cypress, Lavender, Lemongrass, or helichrysum essential oil.
- Apply the mixture to your face and neck.
- Leave it on for about five minutes and then rinse it off with lukewarm water.

Follow this remedy once daily for several weeks. Note the changes.'

Also include strawberries in your diet to get faster results.

6. Cinnamon Scrub

Another great remedy for sagging skin is cinnamon. It helps accelerate collagen production, which is essential for firm, tight skin.

- Mix one teaspoon each of cinnamon powder and turmeric powder with enough olive oil to make a paste.
- Add several drops of lavender, cypress, frankincense, patchouli or carrot seed oil.
- Then mix in one-half teaspoon of sugar or salt.
- Gently scrub your face and neck area with this paste for a few minutes.
- Wash your face with lukewarm water.
- Use this natural scrub once or twice a week.

ADDITIONAL TIPS

- To tighten your skin, perform facial muscle exercises twice daily.
- Exercise regularly for a well-toned look.
- Exfoliate your skin once to twice a week to get rid of dead skin cells.
- Get eight hours of beauty sleep each night.
- Quit smoking and limit your alcohol intake; cigarette smoking and alcohol speed up the aging process.
- Avoid soaps, lotions, creams containing harsh chemicals.

- Colon Cleanse regularly as well as your liver
- Use chemical-free cosmetic products designed for your skin type.
- Avoid refined sugar and highly processed junk food
- Eat lots of fresh fruits and raw vegetables to keep your body nourished.
- Take vitamin C, vitamin E and MSM (methylsulfonylmethane) supplements. If taking medication, check with your doctor first.
- Keep The Skin Hydrated and smooth by drinking an ample amount of water throughout the day.

CARRIER OILS

All the carrier oils have lubricating properties. For some of them to maintain a longer shelf life and to avoid rancidity, it is best to refrigerate them after opening.

Jojoba Oil Moisturizes mature and dry skin, high resistance to rancidity — softens and regenerative value, able to penetrate the skin rapidly; healing inflamed skin (eczema, psoriasis, dermatitis); controls acne, oily skin and scalp. It has an indefinite shelf life stored at room temperature; high in antioxidants.

Avocado Oil (Moisturizes, regenerates and softens the skin and hair; contains protein and vitamins A, D and E) – good for dry skin. May help to restore and maintain skin tone and elasticity; prevent wrinkles and guard against the sun.

Hazelnut Oil lubricates and nourishes all types of skin; it tones and tightens the skin and helps to maintain firmness and elasticity; strengthens capillaries and encourages cell regeneration; beneficial for skin disorders such as dermatitis, eczema and psoriasis. Refrigerate after opening.

Hemp Oil high levels of both EFA's and GLA, a very balanced vegetable oil; anti-inflammatory actions benefitting skin disorders like dermatitis, eczema, itching, redness and swelling; helps with arthritis, backaches, joint problems, rheumatism and sciatica. Best refrigerated good up to 2 months.

Sesame Seed Oil is a facial oil that is beneficial for all skin types. It is very beneficial for eczema, psoriasis and premature aging skin. It also helps to promote healthy skin balance.

Olive Oil a facial oil for all skin types. It is beneficial for both skin and hair. Olive oil soothes, heals and lubricates the skin. Due to its rich antioxidants, it is very moisturizing and rejuvenating to the skin. (See section on Olive oil) Simply rub olive oil with a few drops of your favourite essential oil.

Almond Oil (Rich in mixed tocopherols vitamin E) – good for oily skin and smoothes dry skin, relieves itchiness; contains naturally occurring vitamins B1, B2, B6 and vitamin E. Excellent in protecting the natural beauty of skin and as a massage oil, it promotes a clear, young-looking complexion, and relieves muscular aches and pains.

Apricot Oil high in vitamin B17 and polyunsaturated fatty acids. Excellent for facial massage; benefits all skin types, it is very rich and nourishing, particularly in vitamin A and easily absorbed because of its texture.

Sea Buckthorn Oil Sea Buckthorn is reputed to be one of the best sources of natural antioxidants due to the high content of Vitamin C. It also contains a natural source of Vitamins A, E.

This oil has been getting more in the spotlight – it can effectively combat wrinkles, dryness, and other symptoms of aged skin. It can also be used to promote healing of burns, prevent sunburn when combined with a cream base with essential oils, used for eczema and small cuts or wounds. Furthermore, it has natural UV protection.

- **Wrinkles, Fine Lines and Age Spots**
  Due to its rich carotenoid and fatty acid content, sea buckthorn oil penetrates into the skin and provides an external supply of nutrients that keeps the skin supported and nourished.

- **Heals aged and dry skin**
  Regular application moisturizes and heals dry, parched skin.

- **Anti-aging**
  Regular application of sea buckthorn oil reduces signs of ageing, wrinkles and fine lines. It improves the regeneration rate of epidermal cells. Epidermis is the outermost layer of skin.

- **Relieves eczema, rosacea and acne**
  Combine sea buckthorn oil diluted in aloe vera gel and apply on eczema lesions. Will provide relief from the itching and scratching sensation and also promotes healing.

- **Rosacea**
  It combats rosacea, the excessive redness on skin due to its anti-inflammatory power. Acne—Sea buckthorn may be helpful in reducing the redness of acne pimples and diminishing their size over time.

Camelia Oil is currently making waves in the beauty arena, called tsubaki oil in Japanese. It has been popular in Japan for thousands of years as a traditional moisturizer. Its beautifying benefits are starting to gain more popularity on a global scale.

- Camellia Seed Oil is an excellent anti-oxidant and has properties that are very similar to Jojoba oil. Camellia oil easily penetrates skin without clogging pores, nourishing the skin with approximately 82% of its fatty acids which are composed of Oleic fatty acid (Omega-9), polyphenols, vitamin E, and even plant collagen and proteins.

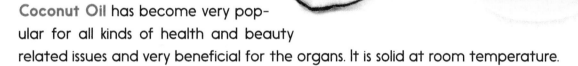

- Camelia protects the skin from free radical damage – **one of the best kept secrets in the cosmetic and hair care industry**. It also has a long healthy shelf life.

Coconut Oil has become very popular for all kinds of health and beauty related issues and very beneficial for the organs. It is solid at room temperature.

- It acts as an effective moisturizer on all types of skin, including dry skin.
- Coconut oil is a safe solution for preventing dryness and flaking of skin. It also delays the
appearance of wrinkles and sagging of skin, an anti-aging oil.
- Coconut oil also helps in treating various skin problems including psoriasis, dermatitis, eczema and other skin infections.
- For that exact reason, coconut oil forms the base ingredient of various body care products like soaps, lotions and creams that are used for skin care. It is used to create a barrier on the skin.
- Coconut oil also helps to prevent premature aging and degenerative diseases due to its well-known antioxidant properties.

  – **Liver**:
  Coconut oil contains the presence of medium chain triglycerides and fatty acids that help in preventing liver diseases. These substances are easily converted into energy when they reach the liver, thus reducing the work load of the liver and also preventing accumulation of fat.

  – **Kidney**:
  Coconut oil helps to prevent kidney and gall bladder diseases. It also helps to dissolve kidney stones.

- **Pancreatitis**:
  Coconut oil is also believed to be useful in treating pancreatitis.

- **Stress relief**: Coconut oil is very soothing to use in massage and hence it helps in reducing stress. Coconut oil applied to the head, followed by a gentle massage, helps to eliminate mental fatigue.

Argan Oil a very rare and precious oil which has been used for thousands of years by the Berber tribes of Morocco enhancing the beauty of Moroccan Women. Its secret properties are now being discovered in other European countries.

- It is rich in freulic acids, eight essential fatty acids, carotenoids, anti-oxidants, sterols, saponins and polyphones and very high levels of vitamin E which is essential for the skin. It even contains Squalene which has been reported to protect against skin cancer.
  - Excellent skin moisturizer to hydrate and soften skin.
  - Anti-Aging – gives skin a youthful glow and reduces the visibility of wrinkles.

Argan Carrier Oil is used in the manufacture of soaps, creams and shampoos. It is used for massage, facials and as an ingredient in anti-aging creams and even aftershave lotion for men. Used for stretch marks, eczema, chicken pox, acne, psoriasis, scars, inflammation, arthritis and joint pain massage.

Black Currant Seed Oil can be used externally as it is generally taken internally. It is an anti-oxidant and protects the cells from free radical damage. Also is a powerful anti-inflammatory.

- It helps to increase elasticity in the skin, and can be used to protect and nourish skin tissues preventing chronic skin conditions such as dermatitis and eczema.
- It can also reduce excessive dryness of the skin and to slow premature aging. Black currant seed oil can be added to skin preparations and cosmetics such as face creams, moisturizers and body lotions.

Tamanu Oil is an exotic and luxurious fatty oil. Tamanu oil is indigenous to Tahiti and south East Asia. Tamanu Oil is a natural nut oil that is extracted from the nut kernels of the Tamanu Tree.

- It possesses significant antimicrobial qualities and can be applied to cuts, scrapes, burns, sun burns, relieves insect bites and stings. It can be applied directly to the skin or blended with other carrier oils for massages.

- Tamanu oil has the unique ability to promote the formation of new tissue, thereby accelerating wound healing and the growth of healthy skin (anti-aging) and has anti-wrinkle qualities.
- Moisturizes, nourishes and repairs the epidermal cells of dry and damaged skin.
- It possesses anti-inflammatory, anti-neuralgic, antibiotic and antioxidant properties.
- Reduces scarring, anti acne and possesses anti viral properties.
- Has antibiotic, antibacterial, anti-fungal and anti-coagulative properties

SPECIAL CARRIER OILS

Borage oil (Borago officinalis) and Evening Primrose oil (Oenothera biennis) are rich (contain high levels) in gamma-linolenic acid (GLA), one of the fatty acids involved in collagen production.

Borage Oil
Borage is known to penetrate the skin easily, benefiting all skin types including skin allergies, dermatitis and inflammation. It is especially beneficial for dry, dehydrated, mature and aging skin. It is also recommended for hormonal imbalances, menstrual, menopausal and pre-menstrual. It is also used for arthritis, circulation, diabetes, obesity, depression, ADD (Attention Deficit Disorder), ADHD (hyperactivity) and liver complaints.

Evening Primrose Oil
Evening Primrose Oil promotes healthy skin and skin repair, and is very helpful for eczema, psoriasis and dermatitis. Like Borage Oil, it is highly beneficial for dry and premature aging of the skin; also used for hormonal imbalances.

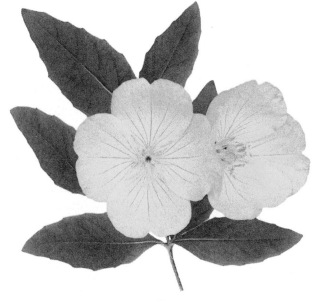

SUMMARY: RECOMMENDED LIST OF BASE OILS FOR AYURVEDIC SKIN TYPES BELOW

(courtesy of Raichur/Cohn & Sachs)

DRY SKIN (VATA)	SENSITIVE SKIN (PITTA)	OILY SKIN (KAPHA)
Avocado	Almond	Almond
Olive	Apricot kernel	Apricot
Almond	Olive	Safflower
Sesame	Borage	Jojoba
Rice Bran	Evening primrose	Evening Primrose
Jojoba	Hazelnut	Sunflower Oil
Hazelnut	Argan	Camelia
Borage	Tamanu	
Evening Primrose		
Camelia		
Sea Buckthorn		
Coconut		

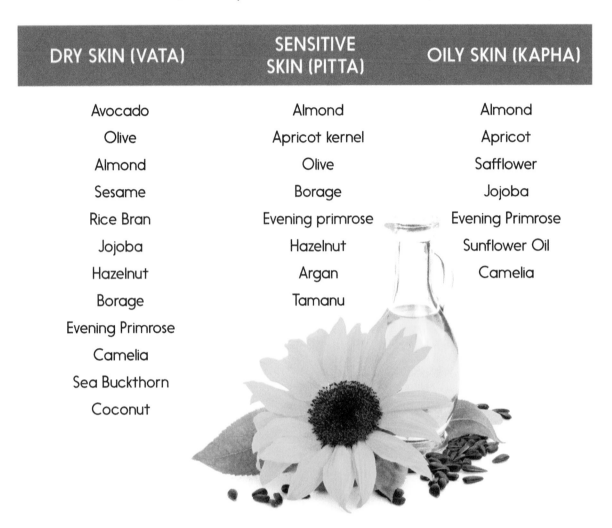

CREATE & BLEND YOUR OWN

Moisturizing Facial Oil
- To your carrier oil of choice, add 15–25 drops of essential oil of choice to
- 15 ml. base oil; unless you are following a specific recipe for wrinkles.
- Mix 2–3 drops of face oil with 4–6 drops of floral water in palm of hand. Stir 3 x clockwise
- Apply on skin.

Special Oils For Your Skin Type

Dry Skin – does not produce enough oil, tends to look dry and dull, and is prone to premature aging.

Oily Skin – produces too much oil, looks greasy and shiny.

Balanced or Normal Skin – distributes skin oil evenly, not too dry or oily.

ESSENTIAL OILS RECOMMENDED FOR DRY SKIN

- Carrot Seed
- Frankincense
- German Chamomile
- Palmarosa
- Sacred Frankincense
- Cedarwood
- Rose
- Sandalwood
- Patchouli
- Jasmine
- Thyme
- Geranium
- Clary Sage
- Myrrh

ESSENTIAL OILS RECOMMENDED FOR OILY SKIN

- Roman Chamomile
- Juniper
- Lavender
- Geranium
- Cypress
- Lemon
- Orange
- Frankincense
- Ylang Ylang
- Rosemary
- Helichrysum
- Lemongrass
- Patchouli
- Rosewood
- Clary Sage

ESSENTIAL OILS RECOMMENDED FOR BALANCED SKIN

- Geranium
- Lavender
- Rose
- Ylang Ylang
- Myrrh
- Lemon
- Frankincense
- German Chamomile
- Sandalwood
- Blue Cypress

A summary of essential oils based on Ayurvedic's skin type is also presented below (Raichur/Cohn, 1997. See book for complete details).

AYURVEDIC'S SKIN TYPE — ESSENTIAL OILS

Essential Oils for Dry Skin (Vata)
(Oils that are sweet, warming, calming, hydrating)

Geranium, sandalwood, lemon, bergamot, chamomile, cypress, frankincense, orange, rose, ylang ylang, jasmine

Essential Oils for Sensitive Skin (Pitta)
(Oils that are sweet, cooling, soothing, hydrating)

Vetiver, ylang ylang, sandalwood, chamomile, cardamom, fennel, frankincense, geranium, lavender, patchouli, rose, spearmint, jasmine

Essential Oils for Oily Skin (Kapha)
(Oils that are pungent, warming, stimulating, drying)

Basil, patchouli, rosemary, sage, peppermint, ginger, lavender, bergamot, clary sage.

COMBINATIONS FOR WRINKLES

(Recipes excerpted from Desk Reference Guide, Essential Science Publishing)

Formula 1
- 1 drop Frankincense
- 1 drop Lavender
- 1 drop Lemon
- Apply day and night.

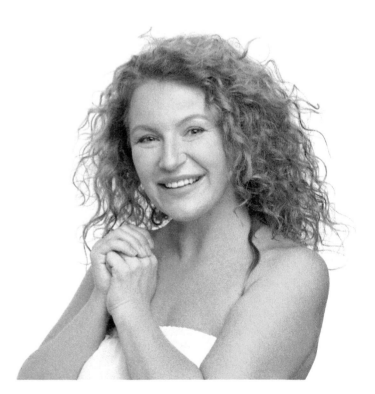

Or Formula 2
- 2 drops Patchouli
- 3 drops Lavender
- 4 drops Geranium
- 6 drops Rosewood
- Mix in 1 oz. of V-6 oil or Jojoba oil. Apply.

Or Formula 3
- Frankincense with Gentle Baby

Or Formula 4
- Add 10 drops Frankincense to Sandalwood Créme

Or Formula 5
- Add 15 drops Gentle Baby oil to 15 ml. carrier oil of choice

Or Formula 6

- 5 drops Sandalwood
- 5 drops Helichrysum
- 5 drops Geranium
- 5 drops Lavender
- 5 drops Frankincense
- Mix with Satin Body lotion. Apply to skin.

Special Facial Oil

- 30 ml. Rosa Rubiginosa (rosehip seed oil)
- 7 drops Carrot Seed,
- 7 drops Frankincense or Geranium,
- 6 drops Rose,
- Mix and apply day and night.

MORE FORMULAS

Over 40

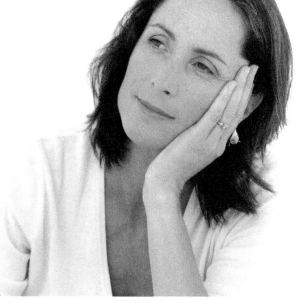

- 10 drops Neroli
- 10 drops Lavender
- 10 drops Frankincense
- 2 drops Rosemary
- 10 drops Fennel
- 3 drops Lemon
- 10 drops Carrot Seed
- 10 drops Evening Primrose Oil

Mix in 30 ml. Hazelnut, apricot or almond oil.

Restore Skin Elasticity	Use Rosewood, Lavender, Carrot Seed or Ylang Ylang with Lavender
Regenerate Skin	Use Geranium, Myrrh, Spikenard, Helichrysum, Rose or Rosewood
Prevent and Retard Wrinkles	Sage, Lavender, Spikenard, Myrrh and Patchouli
Premature Aging of the Skin	Apply Frankincense, Helichrysum, Myrrh or Ylang Ylang or Patchouli on location neat or diluted.

FOR TECH NECK TIPS

Here are some Tips that you can do on a daily basis that will make a huge difference. Remember that the skin on your neck is just as delicate as that found around your eyes, and is two times thinner than that of the rest of the face.

Place your phone more in front of you, if you can so that you are not constantly bending, looking down. Try to use head-phones as much as possible.

Massage your neck daily as you do your face: It is an extension of your face.

1. Use one of the high anti-oxidant carrier oils—like Argan, Tamanu, Sea Buckthorn, Almond, Hazelnut, Rosehip Seed Oil or Black Current Seed Oil—by filling a 15 ml bottle 3/4 full – can also mix 2 of the carrier oils together

2. Add 10 – 15 drops of any of these essential oils and can combine 2–3 of them into the bottle of your carrier oil.

   - Copaiba
   - Blue Cypress
   - Lavender
   - Helichrysum
   - Patchouli
   - Clary Sage
   - Lemongrass
   - Cypress
   - Myrrh
   - Vetiver

3. Drop several drops of your mixture in the palm of your hand- spritz or add a few drops of water and mix together

4. Apply to the neck and Massage by starting under your chin and massage upwards toward the back of your ears. Repeat several times- at least 7 x. Do this 3 x a day for best results.

   Apply your moisturizing cream last – massaging upwards from under chin

   OR

   Use the special neck treatment mentioned earlier:

Blend:

- 10 drops Rose
- 7 drops Clary Sage
- 10 drops Lemon
- 20 drops Carrot Seed Oil
- Add in one teaspoon evening primrose oil.

Massage well into the neck. Leave on for 10 minutes, then wipe off excess.

FOR SPECIAL EYE PROBLEMS

MORE EYE TIPS: PUFFY EYES

Puffy Eyes can be caused by a series of issues: crying, lack of sleep, eye strain, allergies, eating salty foods; also caused by hypertension, liver and kidney problems, poor elimination, low digestive fiber, water retention, menstruation and hormonal changes, candidiasis, parasites. Avoid alcohol and smoking (See Appendix H for traditional Japanese Face Diagnosis).

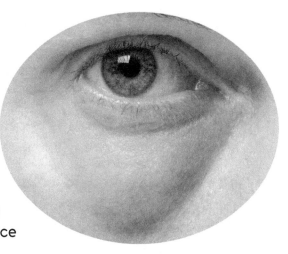

- One of the fastest ways to reduce puffiness around the eyes is with a glass of ice water and four metal spoons. Chill the spoons in the ice water (with 1 tablespoon **witch hazel, plus 2 drops each of fennel and German chamomile)**. Place a spoon over each eye. Replace with cooler spoons when spoons become warm, or

- Wrap 2 steeped tea bags of chamomile or regular black tea or green tea which is high in antioxidants—let them cool, squeeze excess water then lay cooled bags over closed eyes for 2 to 5 minutes, or

- Apply cotton pads dipped in witch hazel or celery juice. Place on closed eyes for 20 minutes, or

- Slice raw potato and place over eyes; relieves puffiness and clears eyes. Can also apply cool cucumber slices over the eyes for 10 to 15 minutes.

- Avoid rich night creams around the eyes at night as the skin under the eyes is extremely delicate—the oil gets trapped and causes puffiness.

- One Indian home remedy for puffy eyes is the application of a compress of a weak solution of sea salt and water. The salt draws water away from the tissues. Rinse eyes with cool water afterwards.

- V. Worwood recommends essential oils of German chamomile, lavender, fennel, carrot seed, lemon, Palmarosa or rose to be mixed with hazelnut or almond oil and applied around the eye area (not on eyelids). Gently massage eyes.

- Make an eye compress with lavender or chamomile (both oils ease inflammation and sore muscles). Add 4 drops lavender or chamomile oil to a cup of cool water. Dip a soft cloth in the water, wring it out and place the cloth over closed eyes for 3 to 5 minutes.

- Use aloe vera gel under the eyes —or vitamin E which is also high in almond oil

- Use Chia gel by mixing: To 1 tablespoon of Chia seeds, add about 3 tablespoons or more of room temperature water into a glass bowl. Add 1 drop German chamomile essential oil.

   Now leave the seeds to soak the water for 25 or 30 minutes or longer. When it becomes a gel, it's ready to use. You can apply directly to the area surrounding your eyes to help repair the skin.

   The Omega 3 fatty acids in the Chia will help reduce the puffiness and help to smooth out fine wrinkles.

MORE SPECIAL TIPS:

Add dandelion tea or tinctures several times daily in your diet (as a natural diuretic to eliminate excess fluid).

- In the Oriental system, puffiness is due to a kidney imbalance.
- Add 1,000 mg. vitamin C a day and vitamin B-6.
- Eliminate salty and allergenic foods, and increase dietary fiber.
- Drink warm/hot water first thing in the morning to help flush the kidneys.

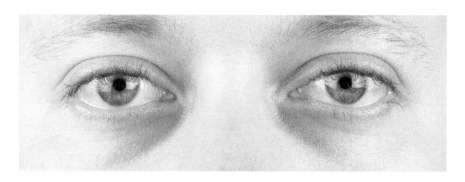

Dark Circles

Dark Circles can also be caused by lack of sleep or staying up late at night, fatigue, illness, allergies, anemia, poor circulation, parasites, hormonal imbalances, menstrual disorders: poor dietary indiscretions and overconsumption of fried/frozen/foods and canned beans, peanuts.

Avoid excess consumption of salt that facilitates fluid retention and causes puffiness and dark circles.

Another tip: Properly clean the eye area in removing makeup to prevent fat from accumulating—avoid harming this delicate area.

- One of the most popular, simple and effective remedies to remove dark circles is the use of **almond oil**. Very simple to do by applying almond oil around your eyes and leaving it overnight. Wash if off gently after waking up in the morning.

- **Cucumber**: This vegetable is one of the most commonly used natural ingredients which reduce dark circles. Its astringent and lightening properties work to reduce the darkness around the eye area, thus increasing blood flow and reducing the puffiness

- **Cold compress** also helps treat dark circles and eye puffiness. Can use an ice bag, cloth dipped in cold water, or a frozen spoon. Simply dab anyone of these near the eyes. This will help to instantly reduce the appearance of dark circles.

- **Chamomile** helps to minimize dark circles by constricting the blood vessels. Place a steeped chilled chamomile tea bag under each eye for 10 to 20 minutes, or use chamomile oil as a compress. Soak cloth or cotton pads in a cup of cool water mixed with 4 drops chamomile essential oil.

- **Tomato juice** is highly effective for treating dark circles. Easy to prepare a mixture: use 1 teaspoon of fresh tomato juice, ½ teaspoon of lemon juice, a pinch of turmeric and gram of Chia powder.

Apply it gently under the eye and leave it for ten minutes and then rinse it off.

Soak cotton pads in witch hazel and lay them on the skin under closed eyes for 20 min., or

- Soak cotton pads in rosewater or cold milk, place over closed eyes for 5 to 10 minutes.

- Apply raw potato compresses over eyes for 15 minutes every second day. Apply almond oil if skin under eyes is dry.

- Apply sliced apples (rich in potassium, vitamins B and C and tannin – which all assist to eliminate dark circles) on each eye for 10 minutes (Bharadwaj, 2000).

- Another recipe given by Monisha Bharadwaj in **Indian Beauty Secrets** is to combine mint, almond oil and honey. Crush 5 fresh mint leaves with a little water. Strain the juice and add to 1 teaspoon almond oil and 1/2 teaspoon honey. Stir and apply a tiny amount under eyes before bed.

Crow's feet and Fine Lines

Crow's feet—fine lines can be caused by anxiety, stress, emotional disharmony, water retention, sun, poor lighting, over work and alcohol.

1. Gently massage eyelids at bedtime with almond or olive oil and a few drops of rose, blue cypress or sandalwood essential oils.

2. Apply witch hazel or sandalwood mixture with water as a toner around the eyes to delay the onset of crow's feet.

3. Apply a small amount of almond oil on middle fingertip. Gently massage around both eyes starting at the inner part of your eyebrows, glide over eyebrows towards temples and underneath the eyes – gentle pressure along the cheek bones. Circle the eyes 30 times, once a day. Wipe off any excess oil.

4. Dip cotton pads in rosewater, lie down and place over closed eyes for 10 to 15 minutes to relieve bloodshot eyes. Can also use raspberry leaf tea – soak cotton pads or soft cloth in cool tea to make a compress. Apply over closed eyes for 10 to 15 minutes.

5. Use eye bright herbal tea externally as an eye wash, and internally to strengthen the eyes.

6. Protect eyes by wearing sunglasses outdoors.

For Eye Strain and To Improve Vision
Take frequent eye breaks when reading or working for extended periods of time.

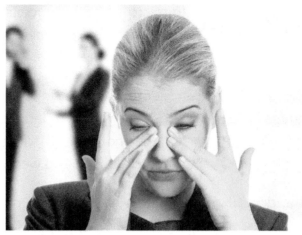

- Rub 2 acupressure points below the collar bone on either side of the sternum, while holding the navel simultaneously. Move the eyes circularly both ways. (Brain Gym)

- Palming every hour—cover closed eyes with your palms to exclude all light, relax a few minutes to experience "no light." Helps to relieve eye strain and bloodshot eyes. For further relaxation, add 1 drop of lavender oil to palms, rub together and then palm eyes.

- Do rapid eye blinking in quick succession about 10 times, up to 5 times a day.

- Extend your right arm straight in front of you. Swing it up and circle to the right (creating a sideways figure 8) then to the left. Follow arm with your eyes without moving your head. Repeat with other arm. Do several times daily. (Brain Gym)

Use Clary Sage to:
- To soothe your eye problems, soak a clean cloth in a mixture of warm water and a few drops of clary sage oil. Afterward, press over both eyes for 10 minutes.

- Called Focusing—look at a distant object, and then slowly bring your gaze to something close at arm's length away. Repeat focusing far to near, near to far; helps eyes to adjust to change. (Brian Gym)

- While sitting on a chair, drop your head between the knees—try to reach for the floor with the crown of your head. Hold for 5 minutes—modified Yoga exercise for improving vision. (Bharadwaj, 2000)

ORIENTAL ROOTS MASSAGE AND ACUPRESSURE

According to the Chinese masters, wrinkles are the result of habitual smiling, concentrating, worrying and squinting. Deeper wrinkles as seen around the nose, mouth, eyes and forehead are due to micro-spasms of specific muscle groups. Emotional expressions also cause these muscles to contract—and over time they cause micro-spasms and toxicity to develop within these muscle fibers.

This causes the skin's metabolism to slow down. To the Chinese, the two most abused muscle areas in the body are the face and the back. To state this simply, wrinkles are due to muscular contractions. The Chinese tradition of massage is considered vital to good health, and recommended 2–3 times a week.

The accupoints for facial rejuvenation correspond to neuromuscular motor sites. According to the Chinese 5 element relationship, the lung governs the skin. The lung point is always employed. By applying acupressure and massage over these points, the muscle spasms can be eased and wrinkles disappear. Now we will combine both methods: a) good skin care habits with healthy eating and the essential oils that will also nourish the skin and relax the skin muscles, and b) applying the Acu massage techniques to relax the spasms and create circulation in the skin – now we can maximize the benefits of both systems. Facial wrinkles are caused by spasmed facial muscles due to habitual emotional expressions, negative emotions, stress and toxic build-up.

FACIAL WRINKLES ARE CAUSED BY SPASMED FACIAL MUSCLES DUE TO HABITUAL EMOTIONAL EXPRESSIONS, NEGATIVE EMOTIONS, STRESS AND TOXIC BUILD-UP.

DAILY REMINDERS:

1. Cleanse face of any impurities—morning and evening.

2. Massage essential oils on damp skin. Use toner (floral water) or make your own.

3. Massage face and neck, with upward gentle strokes.

4. Massage around the eyes in a circular direction from the outside corner to inside.

THE ROSE (ROSA DAMASCENA)

5,000 lbs. of rose petals —1 lb. of Bulgarian Rose oil with a frequency of 320 Hz., the highest in the plant kingdom.

The Rose was known as the queen of all flowers, christened by the Greek poetess Sappho. The rose has a rich history in many cultures. Ancient Greeks prized the rose as the flower of Aphrodite, the goddess of love. Early Christians attributed it to the Virgin Mary. To the Arabs, the rose represented the highest spiritual achievement. Ancient Egyptians considered the rose a cure-all.

Bulgarian scientists have demonstrated that rose oil can reduce high blood pressure and heart arrhythmia, plus its value for ulcers, headaches to elevating the Mind and Spirit. Rose oil is a cell rejuvenator, having softening, hydrating and anti-inflammatory effects on the skin. It disinfects and soothes dry, delicate and mature complexions. Rose is suitable for all complexion types.

CHAPTER 12

FACIAL-LIFT HOME SPA PROCEDURE

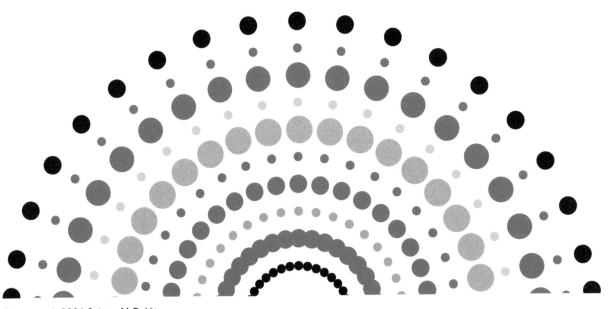

"Inner beauty should be the most important part of improving one's self."
PRISCILLA PRESLEY

DAILY AND WEEKLY REGIMEN

STEP A—CLEANSING

This removes dirt and impurities from the surface of the skin. Use a cleanser to remove makeup and dirt that collected during the day. Worwood reports how the ancient Romans massaged oil into their skin, then scraped it off to remove the dirt. Cleanse daily.

Simple cleansing oils for all skin types

To 1 oz. carrier oil (hazelnut, almond, hemp, jojoba, olive, avocado or sesame – use heavy oil like avocado for dry skin, light oil like almond for oily skin) add 6 to 10 drops of essential oil of choice: Lemon, Sage, Clary Sage, Thyme, Lavender, Rosemary or Geranium. Blend oils and apply to face. Gently wipe off with warm, wet washcloth.

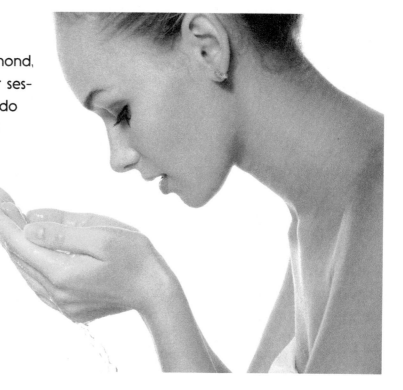

FOR DRY SKIN	FOR OILY SKIN	FOR BALANCED SKIN
• 1 oz. Jojoba	Combine:	• 1 tsp. French green clay or baking soda
• 2 drops Myrrh	• 1 tsp. French green clay powder or baking soda	• 1 tsp. honey
• 1 drop Fennel	• 1 tsp. water	• 1 drop Lavender
• 1 drop Frankincense	• 1 drop Ylang Ylang or Sage, Lemongrass, Cypress, Basil, Cedarwood (slows down oil production)	• 1 drop Rosemary
• 1 drop Patchouli		• Mix in palm of your hand.
• Blend and massage oil into your skin. Wipe with a warm, wet washcloth	• Mix in the palm of your hand.	• Massage into your skin.
OR to	• Massage into your skin	OR to
• 1 oz. Sesame oil, add 1 to 2 drops Rose or Sandalwood, Jasmine and Geranium	OR to	• 1 oz. almond oil, add 1–2 drops Basil, Rosemary or Lemon oil
	• 1 oz. jojoba, Add 1 to 2 drops Lemon and Cypress	• (V. Worwood)

* A rule of thumb in esthetics is that for every night that makeup is not removed, it ages the skin seven days.

STEP B—SCRUBS OR EXFOLIATOR

Apply before bedtime to remove impurities. Exfoliate or use a scrub 2 to 3 times a week.

Use warm water, never hot. In the morning, wash with warm water only. Avoid abrasive scrubs if skin is sensitive.

Avoid soaps: they strip the skin of its protective mantle. Scrubs gently slough off or **exfoliate dead skin cells** that can contribute to blemishes, dryness and wrinkles. Scrubs can help to boost circulation to your face.

1. First splash your face with warm un-chlorinated water.

2. Scoop the scrub onto your fingers and massage all over your face in a circular motion.

3. Rinse your face with warm water. Pat dry.

Extra Gentle Every Day Scrub

Pour 2 to 3 tsp. of baking soda into the palm of your hand. Add 1 drop of Lavender or Clary Sage; add a little warm water to make a paste. Apply and massage in a circular motion.

Ready-made Scrubs

Juniper (from Young Living) for oily skin. This is an exfoliating scrub designed to gently eliminate layer of dead skin cells.

Mint Scrub (from Young Living) for normal skin. Both scrubs can be used as a drying face mask to draw impurities from the skin.

Other Facial Scrubs:

Use cornmeal (blue is finer), flaxseed meal or oatmeal. Add 1/2 teaspoon in the palm of your hand, add water to make a paste; add 1 to 2 drops oil such as Lavender, Ylang Ylang, Geranium or Clary Sage.

All Purpose Scrub

- 1 tsp. blue cornmeal a little warm water

- 1 drop Lavender

- 1 drop Ylang Ylang Mix and apply on face.

- Rinse well.

OR

- 1 tsp. ground almond

- 1 tsp. almond oil

- 1 drop Lemon

- Mix and pat over face.

- Leave for 30 seconds.

Rinse well. Do 2 times a week.

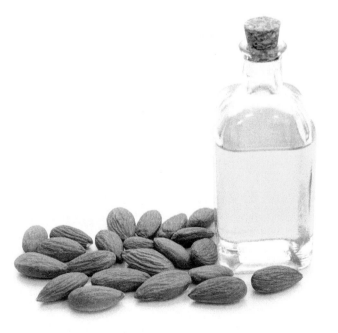

OR

For Dry Skin, add egg yolk to chickpea flour (softens skin) with a teaspoonful of honey and 1 drop of Lavender – spread over the face and neck, wait 20 minutes, then wash off.

To lift graying cells and enliven skin tone. Add 1/2 teaspoon apple cider vinegar, 1 pinch sea salt, 1 teaspoon oat flakes and 1 teaspoon ground almonds with 1 drop Basil oil. Mix Basil, salt and vinegar first.

Chia Seed Scrub

- 1/4 cup coconut oil

- 1/2 tablespoon lemon juice

- 1 T Chia seeds

- 1 drop Lavender or Lemon

- Mix and set for 2 minutes for the mixture to gel.

- Apply and massage — rinse well.

> "To a large extent, your skin's age depends on how well you take care of it."
>
> – UNKNOWN

Skin Brightener Scrub

- 2 T baking soda

- 1/2 mineral water

- 1 drop lemon oil

- Make a paste and apply on face.

- Leave for a minute to dry.

- Wash with warm water.

- Rinse with cool water..

STEP C—MASSAGE FACE AND ACUPRESSURE POINTS (YOUR FACE-UPS)

According to Roberta Wilson, esthetician, aroma therapist and author, facial massage increases circulation to your skin and improves the complexion. This helps bring problem skin into balance.

To the Chinese and Indian Ayurvedic traditions, massage is considered just as essential to health and beauty as a good diet. Massage gives luster to the skin, tones and relaxes the underlying muscles, increases body heat, improves circulation, flushes out waste products and rejuvenates the skin.

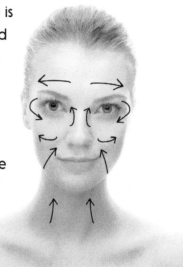

Applying acupressure to specific face points enhances the procedure to produce better results.

To 1 oz. carrier oil, add 6 to 10 drops oil of your choice (e.g. Lemon, Clary Sage or Ylang Ylang) as your face and neck massage oil.

For Dry Skin

- Chamomile, Lavender, Clary Sage*, Cedarwood, Geranium, Myrrh, Jasmine, Rose, Sandalwood or Patchouli ~10 drops of each mixed with 1 oz. carrier oil (Rosemary will stimulate oil production).

For Oily Skin

- Clary Sage*, Lemongrass, Ylang Ylang*, Geranium, Juniper, Lemon*, Orange, Sage, Rosewood,

- Sandalwood or Cypress help to normalize oil secreting sebaceous glands. Add 10 drops to 1 oz. carrier oil.

Balanced Skin

- Rose, Geranium or Neroli, Ylang Ylang*, Cedarwood, Clary Sage*, Lavender, Patchouli, Sandalwood

- Apply appropriate blended oil for your skin type all over face and neck. Follow the pictures:

NOTE: Lubricate well and massage face two times a week. Can be done with a face massager. Repeat steps 4 times.

NOTE: Massage face daily (a mini-massage) in the morning when applying facial oils as your moisturizer.

THE MASSAGE PROCEDURE

1. Begin at the base under the chin and stroke upward to the top of each ear.

2. Start at the jaw and move your hands to the corner of the mouth; to the corner of the nose; cheekbone; then over to the temple to the middle of the forehead.

3. Make a circle from inner corners of the eyes and under your eyes.

4. Massage upper lip outside of the mouth.

5. Stroke forehead upward into hairline.

6. Massage head by gently tapping the head all over, to stimulate the circulation. Rub along the scalp and gently move the scalp over the head. Gently tug on the hair from the roots — helps to relieve muscle tension.

7. End the session with an energy sweep massage. Rub dry hands together for 36 times to increase "chi" energy. Add 1 drop Ylang Ylang or your favorite oil into the palm of your hands. Move your hands over your face, starting from chin upwards to forehead, along the hairline, over the ears and down back to chin. Repeat circular motion 36 times.

NEXT: APPLICATION TO THE ACUPRESSURE FACE POINTS.

Now follow the **acupuncture chart**, apply light pressure and hold for 10 to 20 seconds with a sharp pen like object or auricular probes. If using fingers, rub in gentle, small clockwise circles. Best to be done one to two times a week. See Appendix B for a larger facial chart.

Emotional Tapping Aroma Release: (ETAR) Check Chapter 13 for a simple variation.

*Ylang Ylang especially relaxes facial muscles and releases facial tension that contributes to lines and wrinkles.

STEP D—STEAM (YOUR FACIAL SAUNA)

Steams are an aromatic way to deep cleanse your pores, moisturize your skin and improve circulation to your face. Steams are extremely helpful for seborrhoea and acne problem skin as well as to regenerate mature skin.

Inhaling the aromatics is also beneficial for respiratory ailments, anxiety, colds, flu, head-aches, stress and sinusitis. Steaming is best done once a week. It makes masks twice as effective to rid the skin of impurities. Use oil for your skin type.

FOR VERY DRY OR SENSITIVE SKIN: OR DON'T HAVE THE TIME

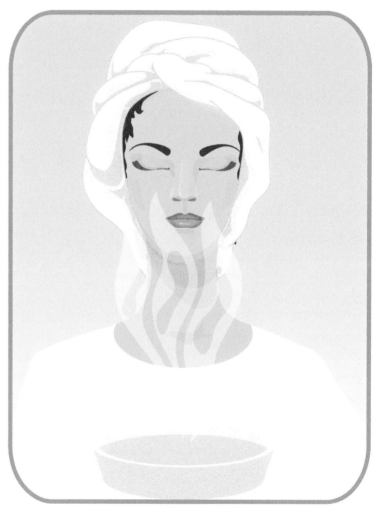

Use hot compress as an alternative to steam. Simply immerse white washcloth in a mixture of hot water with drops of essential oil. Wring out the cloth and apply it to the face. Repeat this process several times. This is a very soothing procedure.

Procedure:

1. Steam after scrub and massaging face.

2. Steam face – drape towel over your head and bowl to catch the steam (take boiling water off the burner) or use a store bought steamer; put your face over the steam about 12 inches from the water, relax for 10 minutes with eyes closed.

3. Rinse with cool water afterwards or massage with ice cold face cloth.

Lavender Steam
Soothes and tones, and gives a rested feel.

- 4 cups warm water

- 6 to 8 drops of Lavender or use Lavender essential water

- Bring 2 cups of water to boil, remove from heat. Add remaining 2 cups with the essential oils. Can also use a professional steamer. Use 1 to 2 drops of oil in water.

Citrus "Fresh"
Leaves skin fresh and thoroughly clean.

- 4 cups of warm water

- 1 lemon, 1/4 inch slices

- 2 drops Tangerine essential oil

- After boiling 2 cups, add lemon; steep for 1 minute, and then add oil and remaining 2 cups of water.

For Dry Skin:
- Add 2 drops of German Chamomile and Rose Oil to a bowl of steaming water.

For Acne:
- Use 2 drops each of Clary Sage, Thyme linalol, Lavender and Chamomile to steaming water. Follow steaming procedure.

STEP E – MASKS

Many choices
Facial masks have many benefits: can nourish your skin, moisturize, rejuvenate, stimulate, as well as cleanse and peel off the outer skin layer. Masks can also clear acne, act as an anti-wrinkle treatment and natural face-lift. Masks are a great way to invigorate your complexion and face tone.

Masks are recommended once a week. Use a cleansing mask first and then follow with a second rejuvenating mask. Agave or Honey Soufflé Mask – tightens pores and gently hydrates your skin (do not use if skin is broken).

Honey Mask

Honey is a powerful natural moisturizer. Great for dry skin.

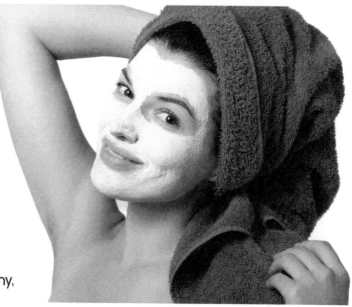

- 1 egg white

- 1 tsp. agave or honey

- 2 drops Lavender oil

- Beat egg whites until frothy, fold in agave/honey and Lavender.

- Apply mask to face and neck, wait 10 minutes. Rinse with warm water.

- For normal skin, add rosewater to 2 tablespoons of milk powder; mix. Create a paste and apply to face and neck. Wait for 10 minutes.

Banana Honey or Agave Mask

A good for all skin types, and leaves face softer and moisturized. Add 1 to 2 drops **Lavender, Ylang Ylang** or your oil choice.

- 1 ripe banana

- 1 Tbsp. honey or agave

- Mash together. Apply to face and wait 10 to 15 minutes.

- Rinse with warm water.

Wrinkle Reduction Mask:

Chinese beauties like to make face masks with egg whites to keep their facial skin glowing and taut. Egg whites are astringent helping to firm skin.

- 1 or 2 egg whites

- 1 drop of frankincense

- Apply the egg whites and let it dry. Rinse it off after 20 minutes using cool water.

Another variation: Firming Mask

- 1 egg white

- 1/4 cup avocado

- 1–2 drops Myrrh, Patchouli, Carrot Seed or Sandalwood essential oil

- Whisk together and massage on the face and neck.

- Leave for 5–10 minutes.

- Remove with warm cotton pad or washcloth, that have been soaked in warm water.

Honey Yogurt Mask

Use Manuka Honey for even more skin benefits.

- 1 T plain yogurt

- 1 tsp of honey

- 1 drop lemon oil

- If your skin is oily, add 1/2 t freshly squeezed lemon or lime juice-one drop lemon essential oil.

- Combine and smooth over your face for 15 minutes.

- Rinse with warm water.

Stevia Extract Mask

- Helps for fine lines and wrinkles

- Softens the skin

- Smoothes skin and wrinkles, for greasy skin; tightens skin

- Heals various skin blemishes, acne, seborrhea, dermatitis and eczema

- Helps cuts and wounds to heal rapidly without scarring

- Apply drops in palm first.

- Apply to face; cover entire face and neck.

- Wait 10 to 15 minutes.

- Rinse with warm water.

Facial Mask Dry/Mature Skin

- 2 tsps. honey or agave

- 1 drop Frankincense

- 1 drop Sandalwood

- Mix above in the palm of your hand and apply to clean skin.

- Relax for 15 minutes.

- Rinse Thoroughly.

Simple Cherry Mask for Dry Skin

- Apply a pulp of fresh cherries to your face at night.
- Leave it on for 15 minutes and then rinse it off.

Relieves dry skin and gives you a beautiful complexion.

Simple Satin Scrub as a mask
Use Juniper (for oily skin) or Peppermint (for normal skin) Satin Scrubs as a face mask.

- Apply and leave to dry.
- Wash off with warm water.

Other Homemade Quick Variations

MASK FOR DRY SKIN	MASK FOR SENSITIVE SKIN	MASK FOR OILY SKIN
Banana or avocado pulp (Raichur/Cohn)	Banana or pineapple pulp (Raichur/Cohn)	Strawberry or papaya pulp (Raichur/Cohn)

Chocolate and /or Cocoa Masks

Dark chocolate has the highest amount of antioxidants – must be 70% or higher cacao

High antioxidant chocolate facial benefits include:

- Cell repair and cell damage prevention. Antioxidants neutralize free radicals and prevent them from damaging cells.

- Dark Cocoa—helps firm & prevent wrinkles, due to its high content in vitamins & in minerals

- Helps to increase hydration, decrease skin roughness, increase defense of UV damage.

Vitamin content:

Vitamins **A, B12, B-complex, D and E**, great for absorption of calcium, tissue growth and releasing energy.

Mineral Content:

Chocolate contains copper, iron, manganese, magnesium and zinc which helps for the promotion of cell growth, the repair of tissue and the absorption of nutrients.

Cocoa is also a **rich source of sulfur**, also known as the beauty mineral, necessary for healthy skin.

Hence eating good quality cacao, a superfood is beneficial too—sulfur is also found in Sulferzyme a product that is found in Young Living!

- 1 tsp. Cacao powder

- 2–3 tsp of warm water

- 2 drops of your favorite oil – Lavender, Geranium, Palmarosa, or Frankincense, or Young Living chocolate prepared mask

- Melt the chocolate

- Apply on face with brush

- Wait 15–20 minutes until it dries.

- Rinse with warm water.

Turmeric Mask

Turmeric face masks are used to rejuvenate skin and are very popular in Ayurvedic traditions. Regular use of turmeric with various combinations of ingredients can soften the appearance of wrinkles and fine lines. A few combinations are listed below- be creative with your choices of essential oils.

Caution: turmeric will stain material – so use a towel or washcloth that you don't mind staining.

- 2 teaspoons turmeric powder,

- ½ cup chickpea flour or Chia seed flour

- Dash of almond oil or coconut oil

- Add 2 drops sandalwood essential oil.

- Add water to above combination to make a paste.

- Apply this mask and leave it until it dries about 15–20 min.

- Wash off with warm water.

Along with the mask—add the chamomile tea bags (after use and cooled down), or 2 cucumber slices or 2 cotton balls soaked in lavender or rose water on your eyes.

Relax for at least 20 minutes, giving your face mask sufficient time to dry and stiffen. Rinse with warm water, gently removing all remnants of your mask. Finally, splash on some cold water on your face and pat dry.

More turmeric masks
For dry skin:
- Combine 1 teaspoon turmeric,

- 1 tablespoon coconut flour or powder

- Add water.

- 1 drop Myrrh, Patchouli, Carrot Seed or Sandalwood essential oil

- Apply for 10–15 min and let dry

- Wash with warm water

For both skin types

- 1/4 teaspoon turmeric powder

- 2 tablespoons coconut flour or chickpea flour (to thicken the paste)

- a few drops of honey

- Add 1 drop of Geranium, Lavender, Clary Sage or Sandalwood essential oil.

For Dry skin

- add an extra 2 tbsp of jojoba, olive, hazelnut or avocado oil

- Leave the mask on for 15–20 minutes.

- Use a warm, wet washcloth that you don't mind staining.

- Rinse off the mask.

Acne skin:

- 2 tablespoons milk or yogurt

- 1/2 teaspoon turmeric

- 1/2 teaspoon sandalwood powder or 2 drops sandalwood oil

- Mix to form a smooth paste.

- Keep for 10–15 min and then wash off

Turmeric mask for oily skin:

- 1/4 teaspoon turmeric powder

- 1–2 drops of lemon oil

- 2 T almond or jojoba oil to form a smooth paste.

- ADD—water to acquire the correct consistency if need be

- Apply and keep for at least 10 min

- Wash thoroughly

Skin Tightening Turmeric/Egg Facial Mask

- 1/3 teaspoon Turmeric powder

- 1 Egg white

- 1 tablespoon Oats or Chia seed powder

- 1 drop of carrot seed, lavender or helichrysum essential oil

- Blend all these ingredients in a bowl.

- Apply the mixture on your face and neck.

- Scrub gently in circular motion.

- Wait for 15 minutes then

- Wash off with cool water.

This mask helps to tighten the sagging skin and helps to retain the younger look.

Skin Firming Formula for Any Skin Type

- Aloe Vera (cut an older leaf from a plant if you have one – provides the best in nutrients – otherwise use 100% aloe vera gel.)

- Rub aloe on face and neck and leave for 20 min. Can sleep with it as well.

- Rinse and apply your moisturizers.

Avocado Face mask

Avocados are a great food that are high in Vitamins A, D, E, proteins, lecithin, beta carotene and more than 20% essential unsaturated fatty acids. All of these nutrients are excellent for the skin. This mask will help for various conditions: **dry skin, eczema, great for reducing age spots, scars, and sun damage.** Avocados contain plant sterols, which help boost **collagen** production and will help to **hydrate and refresh** your skin leaving it with a beautiful, healthy glow.

Avocados have a **natural sunscreen** in them. Avocado oil will add extra moisturizing and sun protection benefits to your homemade sunscreen oil combinations so add a few teaspoons when making your own sunscreen.

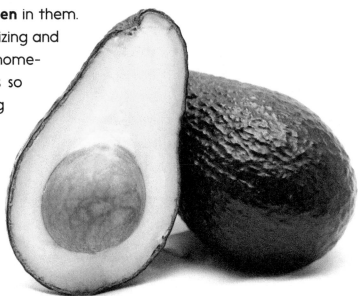

Add Lavender oil (a major cell regenerator that is also great for clarifying skin) or Clary sage. Other essential oils that can be added instead: Carrot Seed, or Geranium

- 1 ripe avocado

- 20 drops lavender essential oil or Geranium

- 1.5 tbs. honey or Agave

- 1 tbs. plain yogurt

- Mash your avocado in a glass bowl.

- Add the honey, yogurt, and lavender essential oil to a nice creamy consistency. Apply to your face and leave on for 10–15 minutes.

Can be used on your feet too.

Simple Avocado mask

- Mash your avocado in a glass bowl.

- Add a few drops of your favorite essential oil.

- Apply directly to your face.

- Leave on for 10–15 minutes.

- Wash off with warm water.

Matcha Green Tea mask

Matcha green tea is a much healthier, immune boosting high anti-oxidant tea than your regular green teas as it is the whole tea leaf that has been ground into a powder. Matcha green tea has up to 10 times the antioxidant power due to using the whole leaf.

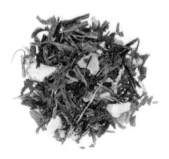 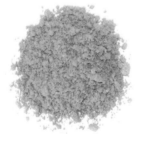 

Research findings indicate that Japanese (not Chinese) green tea contains approximately 100 times more Vitamin C antioxidant power, about 25 times more Vitamin E antioxidant power and is a rich source of Polyphenols.

Recent medical research has concluded that Japanese green tea not only prevents UV skin damage but actually promotes cellular re-growth & even stimulates the repair of Key DNA structures!

ORAC Value

There is a term called the ORAC value that provides a measurement of the anti-oxidant level of a given food. It was developed by the National Institute on Aging in the National Institutes of Health (NIH). The higher the number, the more antioxidant power it has. A website was created to show the ORAC Values www.oracvalues.com that you can easily source to check on foods, or herbs. Matcha shows as having a significant high value.

Matcha Mask #1 (Best for Oily to Normal Skin)

- 1 tsp. Matcha Green Tea powder

- Few drops of Water or Aloe Vera Gel

- 1–2 drops lavender, Geranium or Patchouli, or bergamot

- Combine Matcha Green Tea powder into a small bowl and slowly add water or aloe vera gel with the essential oils. (The thicker the consistency, the better it will stay on your face.)

- Apply to clean face

- Leave on for 15 minutes or longer if desired.

Matcha Mask #2 (Best for Dry Skin)

- 2 tsp. Matcha Green Tea powder

- 1/2 tsp. Organic Coconut Oil, avocado, olive or hazelnut oil

- Few drops of Water

- 1–2 drops of geranium, sandalwood, frankincense, rose or jasmine

- Combine Matcha Green Tea powder into a small bowl and slowly add water and the coconut oil. Mix in the essential oil of choice. (The thicker the consistency, the better it will stay on your face.)

- Apply to clean face

- Leave on for 15 minutes or longer if desired.

Wrinkles, Skin Firmness and Elasticity

Can Green tea help with wrinkles and sagging skin? Some small studies have shown that green tea extract has improved the skin's matrix leading to firmer skin tone.

I believe that combining essential oils with the fatty oils (coconut, olive or hazelnut oil etc) mixed with the green tea would give the best delivery for skin enhancement and improvement. No harm in giving this mask a try!

CHIA SEED MASKS

Chia gel mask for facial redness and scars.
Thanks to the high concentration of omega-3 fatty acids in Chia seeds that help for reducing inflammation.

- Mix 1 Tbsp of Chia seeds with 2-3 Tbsp water and let it set into a gel for 30 minutes. Mix in a few drops of lavender or helichrysum essential oil

- Apply the mixture to red areas and scars. Let it sit for a few minutes before rinsing off with cool water.

Hydrating Chia Mask
This mask is extremely hydrating and can also be used for exfoliation. After you cleanse your skin put this mask on.

- 2 tablespoons of Chia seeds or Ground Chia 1–2 tablespoons of water

- 2 tablespoons of honey

- 1 drop Frankincense, Geranium, Sandalwood, or Lavender or any other oil of your choice

- 1 tablespoon of extra virgin Olive oil, small whisk

- Add the seeds to a bowl of water. Leave the seeds to soak in the water for about 20–30 minutes.

- Once the Chia seeds are of a gel consistency, then add the honey, essential oil and 1 tablespoon of olive oil

- Whisk together and apply on face. Leave for about 15 minutes.

Chia Exfoliation

- 1/2 cup coconut oil

- 1 tbsp lemon juice

- 2 tbsp Ground Chia seeds

- 2 drops Lemon oil or Lavender

- Mix the above ingredients and allow the mixture to set for a few minutes before applying to a damp face.

- Leave on the face for 1–2 minutes before applying circular motion to exfoliate.

- Apply a wet washcloth to remove. Rinse with cool water.

VANILLA MASKS

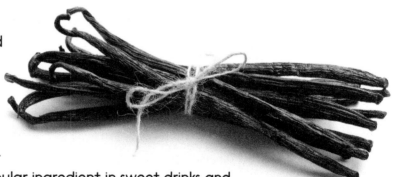

Vanilla beans are sun-dried pods obtained from the orchids of the genus Vanilla. Many are familiar with the amazing sweet vanilla flavor and its fragrance. It has become a popular ingredient in sweet drinks and confectioneries. Vanilla beans are obtained through a labor-intensive process. The antifungal, anti-bacterial properties of vanilla make this a unique food along with its high level of antioxidants and its ability to reduce free radicals in your body. Vanilla possesses both antioxidant and cancer-fighting properties.

The rich antioxidants found in Vanilla help to reverse skin damage caused by free radicals **as well as protect your skin from damage caused by environmental pollutants and toxins**. It helps to slow down signs of aging like fine lines, wrinkles and age spots and soothes irritated skin. It is widely used in the cosmetic industry for its fragrance and for its anti-aging benefits. **Vanilla is a good source of B-vitamins like niacin, thiamin, Vitamin B6 and pantothenic acid which play an important role in the maintenance of healthy skin.**

Raw vanilla beans (powder) infused with organic essential oils imparts a great fragrance besides making your skin smooth and soft.

Vanilla Recipe 1 for a Facial Mask

- 2 tablespoons of vanilla powder

- 2 drops of **Stress Away™ essential oil blend** (contains Vanilla essential oil)

- Enough water to make a paste

- 1 tablespoon of coconut oil

- Mix the ingredients and apply it on your face.

- Leave for 10 minutes or more.

- Rinse off with warm water.

- Follow with a cold water rinse afterwards.

Vanilla's antibacterial properties make it beneficial for the treatment of acne, by helping to cleanse your skin and reducing the occurrence of pimples and acne.

Vanilla Recipe 2 – Skin Irritations

- 2 drops of spearmint essential oil (spearmint essential oil helps to calm and soothe the skin and blocks the growth of bacteria thus helping to minimize the pores)

- 2 tablespoons of vanilla powder

- 3 tablespoons warm water

- Mix and apply to face. Wait 15 minutes.

- Rinse with warm water.

BEST FOR LAST – ORCHID OIL MASQUE

Now when you have completed using the other masks–treat yourself by adding this super-hydrating mask as the very last step. This is quite a treat to experience as well as having a 2nd mask. It also contains vanilla essential oil making it a unique addition for your skin. It will also help to reduce stress and lessen tension in the facial muscles.

This mask is not washed off! If available, purchase the ready–made A.R.T® Beauty Masque by Young Living as it is a premium, orchid-based formula designed to soothe skin and leave it feeling healthier and more radiant.

The virtues of orchid oil were presented in an earlier chapter. Remember: **Orchids store water and rehydrate the skin, making it look younger and healthier.**

If not available, **"Do It Yourself"** method below:

In a small bowl containing 4 oz. of warm water combine 1 tsp. of coconut oil, with 1 spritz of Orchid Serum and 1 drop of these oils:

- Young Living Stress Away™ Essential Oil Blend:

- Copaifera Reticulata™ (Copaiba) Oil,

- Citrus Aurantifolia™ (Lime) Oil,

- Cedrus Atlantica™ (Cedarwood) Bark Oil,

- Ocotea Quixos™ (Ocotea) Oil,

- Lavandula Angustifolia™ (Lavender) Oil

Dip a Facial Mask Sheet (available from Amazon) into the mixture to saturate the mask. Apply over the face and leave for 15-20 minutes.

- The exotic blend of orchid petals in the serum and the pure essential oils by Young Living Company nourishes and fortifies the most delicate areas of the face, helping to promote a more vibrant and youthful appearance. It is super hydrating.

- Do not wash your face afterwards – the orchid oils are like a moisturizing lotion. Suitable for all skin types.

STEP F – TONERS

Toners are used to help cleanse, refresh and to tighten your skin. Best applied every day to a freshly washed face as it allows for better absorption of moisturizers or face oils. You can also use a toner over your face as a mid-day freshener.

1. If you can find hydrosols such as ones sold by Young Living Company in Europe then add it to your regimen as a toner.

   - **Chamomile** essential water – soothes skin irritations and swelling

   - **Clary Sage** essential water – for dry skin, headaches and supports hormones.

   - **Juniper** essential water – excellent to detoxify and cleanse the skin

   - **Lavender** essential water – soothing to the skin.

2. If floral waters are not available—it's easy to **create your own**

   - **Minty Toner** – Peppermint is a naturally antiseptic tonic.

     Add 6 to 8 drops Peppermint essential oil to 1/2 cup witch hazel. Pour into a bottle, mix and apply.

   - **Rosewater** – Create your own. Add 1 to 2 drops Rose Oil in 8 oz. of filtered water. Shake and apply. Stimulating and elevating to the mind; prevents and reduces scarring, softens and sooths your skin.

   - **Normal Skin Toner** – Mix 1 drop Lavender, 1 drop Palmarosa and 1 drop Rosewood in 8 oz. distilled water. Blend well. Apply with cotton ball or spritz on your face.

   - **Dry Skin Toner** – Mix 1 drop Frankincense, 1 drop Rosewood and 1 drop Vetiver to 8 oz. distilled water.

3. Create your own **Sandalwood Toner**: To a 8 oz bottle of witch hazel extract, add 1–2 drops of essential oil of Sandalwood, Roman Chamomile, Rosewood and Myrrh. Lightly mist face and neck.

4. Use **Lemongrass/Rose or Lemongrass/ Chamomile** toner for your face – it degreases and balances skin. To 1 oz. Aloe Vera Juice or Rosewater, add 3 drops Lemongrass essential oil/3 drops Roman Chamomile or Rose. Spritz or lightly mist face and neck.

5. Combine essential oil of your choice with **organic apple cider vinegar.** Add 2 to 8 drops of essential oil (lavender or roman chamomile etc.) to 1 ounce of apple cider vinegar. This helps to minimize age spots, blemishes, fine lines and wrinkles. Relieves skin disorders, calms itching and redness of insect bites, poison ivy and poison oak. It is soothing to eczema, dermatitis, red or inflamed skin.

6. **Simple Toners:** Juicy Grapes – cut and rub over the face and neck, leave for 15 to 20 minutes and rinse off. (Bharawaj, 2000)

7. Spritz your face with mineral water. Better still, Add **1 tsp of Mineral Essence** or any liquid mineral to a 8 oz bottle and fill the rest with water. Add 2–4 drops of Lavender, Geranium or Myrrh essential oil.

STEP G—MOISTURIZER/FACIAL CREAMS

Apply oil blends on the face first (Chapter 7).

Then apply your choice of moisturizer creams. Moisturizer creams are not necessarily needed if you use a carrier oil and essential oil blend for moisturizing your face (always on damp skin).

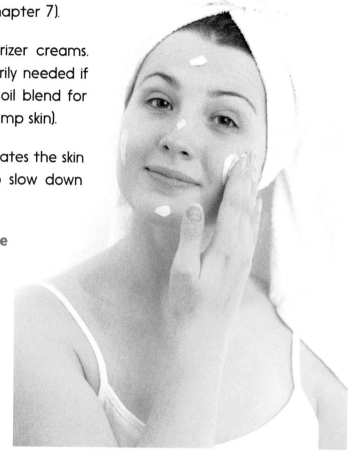

Rose Ointment – feeds and re-hydrates the skin and supplies nutrients necessary to slow down the aging process.

* **Sandalwood Moisturizer Créme** – helps to promote younger, healthier skin.

* **Boswelia Wrinkle Créme** – is a collagen builder. Helps to minimize and prevent wrinkles. Excellent for dry, premature aging skin.

* **Wolfberry Eye Créme** – eases eye puffiness and dark circles. Promotes skin tightening.

To redensify skin, phyto-estrogens are an important ally. Clinical tests revealed an increase of more than 82% in the rate of skin collagen, remodeled facial features by more than 62% and restored skin plumpness by more than 36% with the use of phyto-estrogens. Clary Sage oil is a fabulous one to add.

Phyto-estrogens are the estrogens found in plants that provide low dose estrogens, beneficial for many menopausal symptoms.

NOTE: Use special oil blends after toner, then add moisturizer creams.

FOR THE MEN—AFTER SHAVE SUGGESTIONS

- 2 drops Cedarwood

- 2 drops Cypress 1 drop Elemi

- 1 drop Sandalwood

- Add to 8 oz. of distilled water. Mix and mist the face after shaving. (Excerpt, R. Wilson)

CAN USE Blue Cypress, Cedarwood, Melaleuca, Frankincense or Sandalwood directly on the skin. Apply a few drops in the palm of your hand, rub and apply to face. Spritz face with floral or toner water.

* These creams contain Wolfberry seed oil. They are all combinations from Young Living Company. There are a few more companies today that are providing organic, eco-green moisturizers.

Wolberry seed oil is a costly and unusual ingredient. It's been used by the Chinese living in Mongolia for centuries. It is extracted from the seeds of the Ningxia variety of Lycium barbarum -rich in vitamin E, linoleic and linolenic acids. It is reputed to be outstanding for the skin and is very sought after throughout Asia. It is ideal for nourishing and hydrating the skin, protecting aging skin and adding luster to skin tone.

Orchid Oil Serum
A.R.T.® Renewal Serum from Young Living Company

A.R.T.® Renewal Serum is an intricate blend of exotic orchid petals and essential oils that helps protect and revitalize skin. Similar to the facial masque, these premium ingredients work in harmony to deeply nourish and hydrate the face that helps to create radiant skin.

How to use: After washing thoroughly. Apply small amount of ART Renewal Serum to delicate areas of face 2 times daily. Apply your essential oil combination and moisturizer afterwards.

Another Create Your Own Anti-Wrinkle Formula
Combine in an 8 oz size bottle, 1 tablespoon each of:

- Sea buckthorn oil,

- Jojoba oil,

- Virgin coconut oil,

- Tamanu oil,

With 3–4 drops of each essential oil

- Lavender,

- Vetiver,

- Hawaiian sandalwood

Apply all over face and neck and spritz with your toner to dampen the skin for better absorption

A FULL BODY SKIN TREATMENT

Salt Rubs—A New Experience

Salt rubs are beneficial for energizing and invigorating your skin. It sloughs off dead skin cells, leaves skin moisturized and positively glowing. (Ann Johnson)

1. Buy fine sea salt or Celtic Sea salt. Use one of the recipes below.

2. Shower or bathe so skin is completely wet.

3. Rub small handful of salt all over your body in brisk circular motions ... spend extra time on elbows and heels.

4. Rinse off.

5. No moisturizer needed.

ENERGIZING TONIC FOR YOUR SKIN

- 1 cup fine sea salt

- 2 Tbsp. apricot/almond oil

- 5 to 6 drops Peppermint essential oil or Rosemary, Geranium or Spruce

- Put salt in a bowl, then add oils.

- Mix with hands.

- Store in covered container until ready to use.

STRAWBERRY OR RASPBERRY RUB

- 3 to 4 drops Lemon, Lavender or Rosewood
- 1 cup sea salt
- 3 ripe strawberries/raspberries

Mash together. Mix with hands.

Store in container in refrigerator until ready to use. Good for up to 2 weeks.

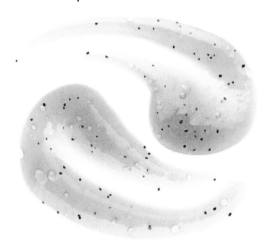

HONEY—YLANG YLANG BODY SCRUB

- 1 tsp honey

- 1 tsp baking soda

- 1 tsp sea salt

- 1–2 drops Ylang Ylang or lavender

- Mix and make a sticky paste.

- Apply over elbows or knees or heels to slough off dead skin cells

SOME BENEFITS OF DRY SKIN BRUSHING:

1. It is one of the best ways to exfoliate dead skin.

2. Dry brushing stimulates your lymphatic system which helps to remove the toxins from your body.

3. Dry brushing also helps to reduce cellulite as it is helping to break down trapped toxins in your body's fat cells.

4. It stimulates your skin so your skin can breathe better and absorb more nutrients. This promotes healthy skin.

"Those who do not find time every day for health must sacrifice a lot of time one day for illness."

FATHER SEBASTIAN KNEIPP

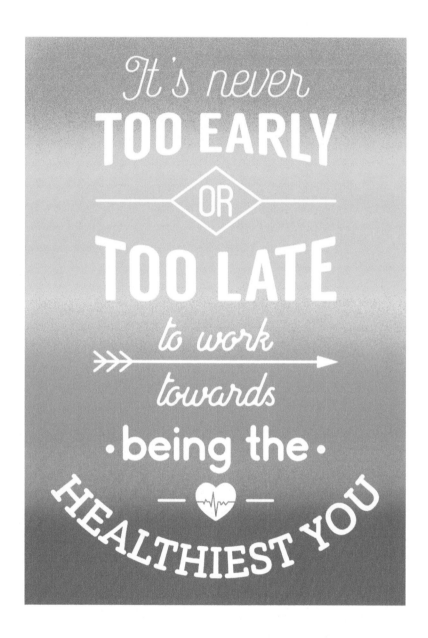

CHAPTER 13

OUR DIVINE MIND: THE AGELESS SOURCE

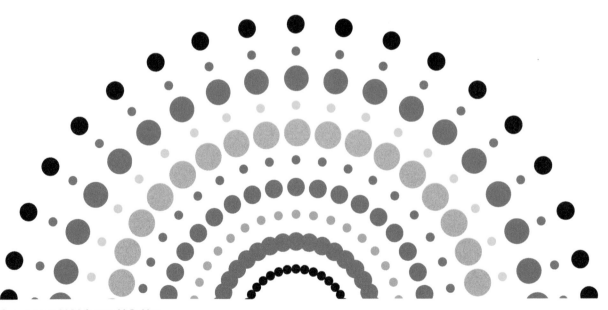

*"How you grow older is your decision...
Don't battle aging when you can dance with life!"*
DR. CHRISTIANE NORTHRUP
"It is not what you do, but how much love you put into the doing."
MOTHER TERESA

We know from Epigenetics how the environment, negative thought and toxic emotions impact every cell in our body-mind. We also know that we can literally change our thoughts and have a direct positive impact on our cells, our skin, our organs. So in summary, as the research suggests, if we change our thoughts and our mood, we can actually change the health and age appearance of our bodies and skin. We can change our programs and our paradigms of aging.

ENERGY PSYCHOLOGY – CREATE BEAUTY FROM INSIDE-OUT

The role of the energy system can also be utilized during a simple facial. Popularly known today as the 'Tapping Solution" by Nick Ortner, many of these same points can be incorporated into a simple routine. My **Emotional Freedom Face-Lift** book outlines a more thorough procedure. Please refer to that book for a more comprehensive routine. Below is a simple everyday routine—the 5 minute version.

SIMPLE – EVERY DAY VERSION

In this case—simply rub and or tap each of the acupressure points by applying the oils to your fingertips first-then apply to the points, while rubbing or tapping say: **(as in step C)**

   a) a releasing statement of acknowledgment, "Even though I feel old . . . I deeply love, accept and respect myself" or "Even though I have wrinkled skin . . . I deeply love, accept and respect myself" or any other version after "Even though I have . . . I deeply love, accept and respect myself"

b) Then repeat the sequence of the points with another essential oil added to your finger tips by adding an affirmative statement—like:

- "I look beautiful".
- "I have healthy skin"
- "My skin is vibrant and regenerates easily", etc.

c) Then apply your moisturizer and toners and repeat your positive statement as you massage the creams over your neck and face. Smile within as you are pampering yourself.

Please check the website for more updates regarding this technique, upcoming videos and the new '**Aroma-firmations**' set.

Look no further for the Fountain of Youth as actress Sophia Loren has found it. She advices us:

"There is a fountain of youth: it is your mind, your talents,
the creativity you bring to your life and the lives of the people you love.
When you learn to tap this source, you will have defeated age."

MY FINAL WORD

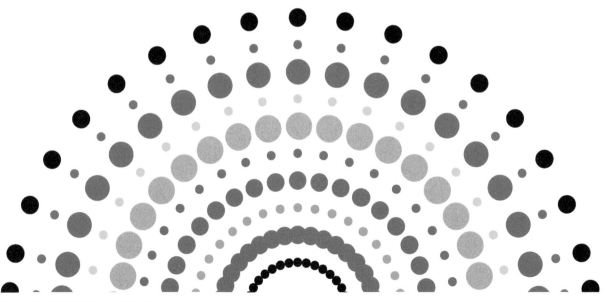

*"Women who live for the next miracle cream do not realize
that beauty comes from a secret happiness
and equilibrium within themselves."*
SOPHIA LOREN

The Ayurvedic ancient wisdom and teachings point out that without happiness, lasting beauty is an unattainable goal. The most important message for being beautiful is not something that is attained externally. It is a body-mind approach where beauty and youthfulness come from within. The purpose of life, according to the Vedic traditions, is the expansion of happiness.

In Chapter two, I presented a section on the holistic paradigm and how the body is a result of one's mental and emotional conditions. What we think and feel manifests in our bodies and shows on our face and complexion. Scientific advances today have ushered in a technology that allows us to visually see the electromagnetic fields (popularly called the "aura" or "chi," "energy" or "prana") that surrounds our bodies, all living organisms and inanimate objects. As mentioned in an earlier chapter, the most advanced whole body imaging device on the market today is called the Gas Discharge Visualization (GDV) Kirlian bio-electrography camera. The GDV camera and its new updated version, the Bio Well, scientifically measures the energy distribution of biological objects. Humanity has now been given a new approach to understanding reality: that we are energy beings, both particles and waves! The energy field is represented by a series of layered colors surrounding the body representing the physical and emotional states of health. The energy field is the cosmic blueprint where illness appears before it manifests in the physical body. In other words, the thoughts and emotions are revealed first.

The awareness that this technology has given to people has been healing in itself. My clients marvel at what I tell them, often sitting in awe from what is revealed. They often ask how do I know so much about them, and I respond *"it's just there in your energy field of information."*

As Martin Luther King so poignantly stated, *"Heavy thoughts bring on physical maladies, when the soul is oppressed, so is the body."* Our thoughts and feelings that we generate dictate and mold the body. Being beautiful and maintaining our youth means creating a beautiful and youthful mind and heart as this will create a beautiful and youthful body. A youthful mind as described by Dr. Deepak Chopra is one that is dynamic, vibrant, curious, enthusiastic, spontaneous, fluid, adaptable, alert, imaginative, playful and lighthearted. The Kirlian camera would display a vibrant, full energy field of an individual who possesses these attributes of a youthful mind. Chopra suggests that in order to grow younger, one must change his/her perception of the body, relinquishing the idea that it's a "bag of flesh and bones."

Instead, he states it's important to experience the body as a field of "vital energy, transformation and intelligence." The youthful mind is also one that makes a conscious choice to stay young and vibrant by retaining one's resiliency, vision, spirit and love of life. Love reverses our biological age—it is the essence of life, our most powerful force that resides in our hearts. Thirty years of research by the Heart Math Institute has shown us that the heart controls and governs the brain. The true seat of the mind is in the heart. It is written in proverbs, *"Whatever a man thinketh in his heart, so shall he be."* Dislike, dissatisfaction, resentment, anger, fear, fear of aging of self only ages the body faster. One study showed that one five minute experience of recalled anger impaired immunity (a dramatic drop in IGA) for over 6 hours!

The latest research on positive emotions shows how DHEA, our youth hormone, was increased by 100% when in a state of gratitude and appreciation. Feelings of appreciation, love, compassion and care generate smooth and harmonious rhythms or coherency. In testing subjects' immune systems, it was shown that when subjects intentionally focused on feelings of care and compassion for five minutes, IGA levels showed to increase by an average of 41% which continued to slowly rise over the next six hours (Childre & Martin).

Compassion is our most precious gift for our immunity, our longevity and beauty. As Raichur/ Cohn states, *"The path to absolute beauty – the path to bliss and wholeness – is not a path of vanity, but of great compassion."*

Learn to "love you." Feel it in your heart and send loving smiles to your face, and internal organs at least 5 to 6 times every day. Look in the mirror and as you apply the oils on your face, rub or tap these few acupressure points and affirm to yourself "I love me" "I am young and beautiful in heart, mind and body."

Become the co-creator of your reality with God. Invite the flow of the divine, the heavenly nectar of love to flow through you. Help to create a world of beauty, peace, love, wisdom, radiance and laughter.

I had fun and laughter playing and creating with the facials and the essential oils. I invite you to have fun too, in exploring the uses, the benefits and the joy in pampering yourself. Relish the Now—the timelessness space!

Be gentle, loving and happy within and you will always be beautiful.

Please note: To assist you with the loving, kind thoughts about yourself, I have created the Aroma-Firming statement plastic card sticker set. It is to go along with your oil application routine. Look for my special Saving Face—'Aromafirmations!' updates that will be posted on the website.

In love, beauty, peace and wisdom,

Sabina M. DeVita

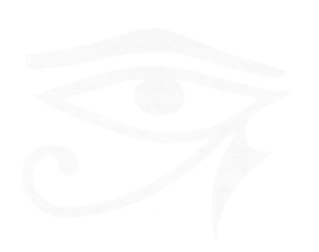

MY FAVORITE QUOTES:

*"The ideals which have lighted my way time after time
have given me new courage to face life cheerfully,
have been kindness, beauty and truth".*
ALBERT EINSTEIN 1879 –1955,
THEORETICAL PHYSICIST

*"If you want to be beautiful, you must first create a
whole and happy inner life, and every part of your body
will rejoice and resonate with that happiness."*
DR. P. RAICHUR/COHN

GDV KIRLIAN BIO-ELECTROGRAPHY PICTURES ARE PRESENTED BELOW, DISPLAYING THE BODY ENERGY DISTRIBUTION OF AN INDIVIDUAL.

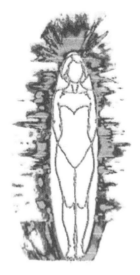

Picture A
In a tired or sick individual, the energy field is weak, thin and disturbed as seen here.

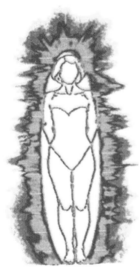

Picture B
The energy field of a healthy individual extends well beyond the physical form, and looks vibrant and colorful.

Enjoy the most pleasant aromatic rejuvenating experience!

Dr. SABINA DE VITA

"Follow your passion to ignite your soul"

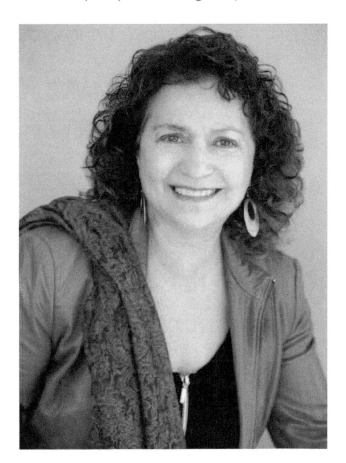

*"The key to health is to have an aromatic bath
and a scented massage every day."*
HIPPOCRATES, FATHER OF MEDICINE,
460–377 B.C.

LOVE—THE GREATEST VIBRATION

Love heals. Love refines.

Love makes you feel safe.

Love brings you closer to God.

Love conquers all fear.

Love makes you young.

Love reverses the aging process.

DEEPAK CHOPRA
(Grow Younger, Live Longer)

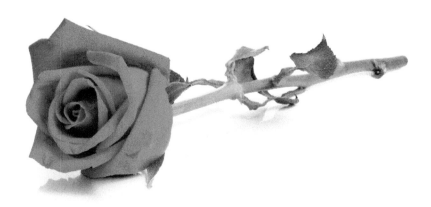

Remember to love, embrace and accept yourself!

YOUR FACIAL MASSAGE PROCEDURE

1. Begin at the base under the chin and stroke upward to the top of each ear.

2. Start at the jaw and stroke upward to corner of mouth to corner of nose, on cheekbone, then over to the temple to middle of forehead.

3. Make a circle from inner corners of the eyes and under your eyes.

4. Massage above upper lip to outside the mouth.

5. Stroke forehead upward into hair line

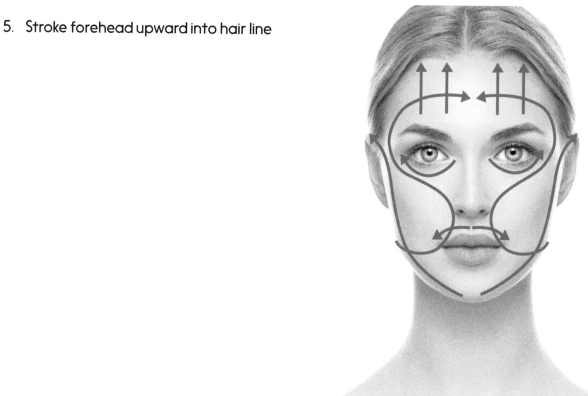

APPENDIX B

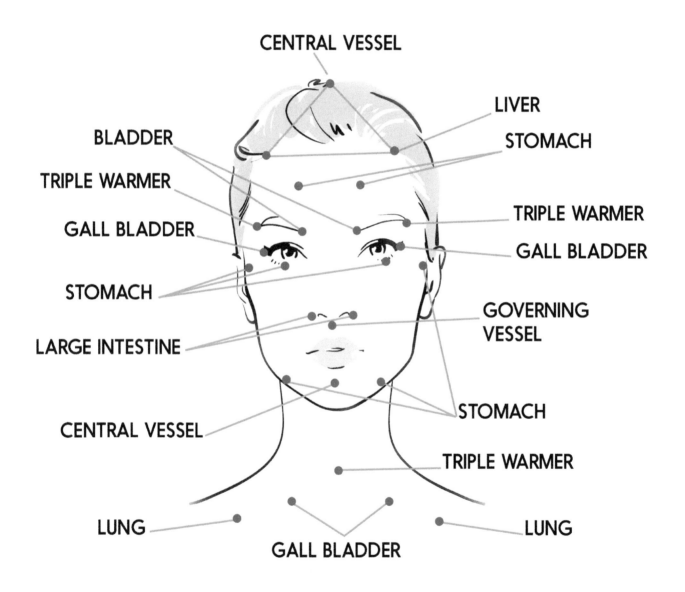

CENTRAL VESSEL

LIVER

STOMACH

BLADDER

TRIPLE WARMER

TRIPLE WARMER

GALL BLADDER

GALL BLADDER

STOMACH

GOVERNING
VESSEL

LARGE INTESTINE

CENTRAL VESSEL

STOMACH

TRIPLE WARMER

LUNG

LUNG

GALL BLADDER

APPENDIX C

YOUR DAILY FACIAL REGIMEN

1. Cleanse face in the morning and before bedtime.

2. Apply toner to refresh your face.

3. Apply essential oil mixture for your skin, then moisturizer cream.

4. Massage face and acupressure points, massage head daily (a mini-massage).

YOUR WEEKLY ROUTINE

1. Cleanse your face.

2. Use a scrub of choice

3. Massage face and use acupuncture face points.

4. Steam your face.

5. Apply mask.

6. Rinse and apply toner.

7. Apply essential oils and moisturizing cream.

8. Spritz with floral water.

IF YOU WON'T EAT IT

1ST VERSE

This old world is getting polluted, we're all convoluted with chemicals.

Endless claims by folks scientific allege they're terrific – the chemicals,

I ain't dumb, I've learned me a thing or two,

Here's what I aim to do now.

Those products cosmetical, if they're not edible just gotta go somehow.

CHORUS

If you won't eat it, then don't wear it, don't rub it on your skin.

What harms the inside will harm the outside and you'll be sufferin'.

If you won't eat it and you won't wear it, well that's a kind of sin. And your bod will know, it will tell you so

And you'll just get sick again.

2ND VERSE

All those creams they say make you youthful, and sexy and beautiful,

How they entice.

Aisles and aisles of grand smelling lotions, and shampoos and potions,

For looking nice.

Best take time to read the ingredients, it's more expedient to

Help you decide before they touch your hide

If you're safe when they're smeared on you.

3RD VERSE

They've got things to keep you from smelling, and sprays for repelling Mosquito bites.

Toothpaste too, and rinse antiseptic. Well, trust this old skeptic,

They're dynamite.

Who can say that it's not diseasing us, while we're appeasing our pride. Well hold all the chemicals, we're staying well because

We ain't doing suicide.

PATTER CHORUS

Titanium, ammonium, glycerin, non-oxynol,

Methyl and colorings, petroleum.

Isoprophyl alcohol, benzoate and glycol,

Chlorine and polyquaternium.

Preservative and acrylates, fluoride, methacrylate,

Aluminum and octylacyrlamide.

Sodium laurel sulfate, dimethacon and sobutane.

Methacrylate and propolene, and chloride.

APPENDIX E

TRADITIONAL JAPANESE FACE DIAGNOSIS WITH WESTERN FACIAL CONCERNS

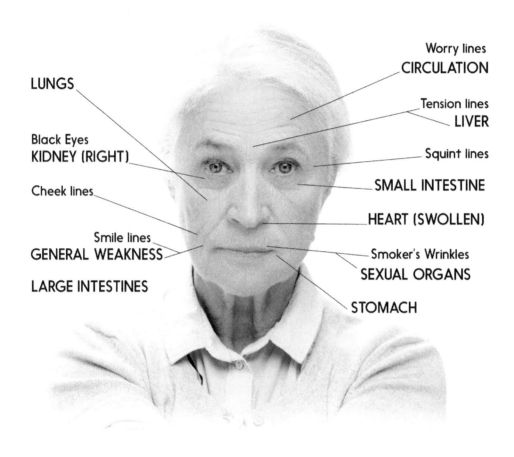

"If you want to be healthy, you have to trade your wishbone for a backbone and get to work."
SOURCE UNKNOWN

"Given the choice of seeing a glowing, youthful face or a dull, wrinkled face when looking into a mirror, I know what I would choose, and now the choice is yours."
JULIAN WHITAKER, M.D.

QUICK ESSENTIAL OIL SKIN CARE REFERENCE CHART

CONDITION	ESSENTIAL OIL	APPLICATION
Acne	Tea Tree, Lavender, Purification, Melrose, Essential Beauty Serum-Acne Prone	Topical
Skin Care:	Facial Scrub (gentle exfoliator) or mix with Orange Blossom Facial Wash	Spread and leave for 5 minutes with hot towel over face. Rinse & apply Sandalwood Crème mixed with any of the above oils
Blisters — 2nd degree burns	Lava Derm spray, Lavender, Spikenard, apply Rose ointment	Topical
Blisters	German Chamomile, Tea Tree, Melrose, Lavender, Purification, Spikenard	
Body Creams	ART Night Reconstructor, Beauty Serum, Tender Tush, Rose Ointment, Sandalwood Moisture Cream, Wolfberry Eye Cream	Topical
Burns — 1st degree burns	Lava Derm spray, Spikenard, Idaho Balsam Fir, Helichrysum, rose, German Chamomile, Lavender, Clara Derm Spray, Gentle Baby, Valor	Topical

QUICK ESSENTIAL OIL SKIN CARE REFERENCE CHART

CONDITION	ESSENTIAL OIL	APPLICATION
Clogged Pores Skin Care:	Purification, Melrose, Inner Child, Orange, Geranium, Cypress, Tea Tree, Lemon, ART Foaming Cleanser, toner	Topical
Dry Chapped, or Cracked Skin	Myrrh, Sandalwood, Lavender, Rose, Palmarosa, Roman Chamomile, Spikenard, Cedarwood	Topical
Itching	Peppermint, Lavender, Patchouli, Oregano, Vetiver, German Chamomile, Aroma Siez, Purification, Melrose, Thieves	Topical
Moles	Oregano, Thyme, Melaleuca, Melrose, Purification	Topical Apply 1-2 drops Oregano 2-3 x a day
Oily Skin	Frankincense, Juniper, Lavender, Lemon, Melaleuca Alternifolia, Sacred Frankincense, Melrose Facial Scrub Mint, Melaleuca soap	Topical
Regenerate Skin	Lavender, Spikenard, Myrrh, Frankincense, Sandalwood, Geranium, Helichrysum, Carrot Seed	Topical

QUICK ESSENTIAL OIL SKIN CARE REFERENCE CHART

CONDITION	ESSENTIAL OIL	APPLICATION
Restore skin elasticity	Sandalwood with Lavender Ylang Ylang with Lavender Patchouli with Lavender, Carrot Seed oil	Topical
Recipe:	6 drops Sandalwood, 4 drops Geranium, 3 drops Lavender, 2 drops Sacred Frankincense- mix with 1 tablespoon high grade vegetable oil – apply 2 x a day	
Sagging Skin	Lavender, Helichrysum, Patchouli, Cypress, Tangerine, Frankincense, Sandalwood, Carrot Seed, Humility, Inspiration, Joy, Blue Cypress, Lemongrass Skin Firming — evening 8 drops Patchouli 5 drops Cypress 5 drops Geranium 1 drop Sandalwood	Special toner for sagging skin Use ART toner, Boswellia Wrinkle cream, Cel-lite 1 drop Neroli, 1 drop Helichrysum— combine with evening Primrose oil or Borage oil, wipe face after cleansing
Scars—Be Gone	Lavender, Helichrysum, 10 drops Helichrysum 8 drops Lemon 6 drops Lavender 5 drops Myrrh 4 drops Patchouli Mix #2 — Helichrysum with Copaiba	Topical Mix formulas and apply

QUICK ESSENTIAL OIL SKIN CARE REFERENCE CHART

CONDITION	ESSENTIAL OIL	APPLICATION
Stretch Marks	Frankincense, Elemi, Spikenard, Geranium	Topical
Wrinkles	Lavender, Thieves, Melrose	Topical
Wounds, Scrapes, Cuts	Carrot Seed oil, Frankincense, Myrrh, Clary Sage, Sandalwood, Gentle Baby, Geranium #1 — 1 drop Frankincense, 1 drop Lavender, 1 drop Lemon to carrier oil — apply #2 — 5 drops Sandalwood, 4 drops Geranium, 3 drops Lavender, 6 drops Frankincense mix & apply	Topical

RESOURCES

INTRODUCTION:

Dr. Christiane Northrup http://www.drnorthrup.com/goddesses-never-age

Somers, Suzanne, *"Breakthrough"* 2008, Crown Publishing Group, Random House Inc. New York

Somers, Suzanne, *"Bombshell"* 2012, Crown Publishing Group, Random House Inc. New York

International Society for Aesthetic Plastic Surgeons http://www. prnewswire.com/news-releases/ the-international-society-of-aesthetic-plastic-surgery-releases-statistics-on-cosmetic-procedures-worldwide-268875081.html

2011 *U.S. News* blog

Health Day Reporter http://www.consumer.healthday.com/senior-citizen-information-31/misc-aging-news-10/pressure-to-look-young-may-be-sending-more-men-to-plastic-surgeons-651011.html

Natural News http://www.naturalnews.com/025278_brain_botox_the.html#ixzz3RByuFbjJ

Huffington Post http://www.huffingtonpost.com/2011/04/14/7-y...)

Mintel http://www.envconsultant.com/men-spending-more-cash-on-skincare-services-at-salons/#sthash.Q5Gb6ETM.dpuf

Cell http://www.cell.com/cell/abstract/S0092–8674(13)01301–9

CHAPTER 1:

Mad Cowboy – (Howard F. Lyman/Glen Merzer: Mad Cowboy - New York: Touchstone eBook, 1998)

Safer Chemicals, Healthy Families http://saferchemicals.org/health-report Epstein – (http://www.preventcancer.com)

Epstein, Samuel, M.D. (1998) *"The Politics of Cancer Revisted"*, East Ridge Press, NY, 770 pp.

Epstein, Samuel, M.D. (2001) *"Unreasonable Risk"*, Environmental Toxicology, Chicago, IL, 204 pp.

Epstein, Samuel, M.D. (2015) (http://www.preventcancer.com/documents/ToxicBeauty_ pressrelease_FINAL.pdf)

Antczak, Stephen & Gina (2001) *"Cosmetics Unmasked"*, Harper Collins Publishers, London 404 pp.

Perricone, Nicholas (2000) *"The Wrinkle Cure"*, Rodale Reach, Rodale, U.S.A., 207 pp.

Dr. Mercola - *Epstein Interview* (http://articles.mercola.com/sites/articles/ archive/2010/04/24/epstein-interview.aspx)

David Suzuki http://davidsuzuki.org/issues/health/science/toxics/ chemicals-in-your-cosmetics

Environmental Working Group — *Skin Deep Guide* www.ewg.org

Safer Chemicals health report - http://saferchemicals.org/health-report

CHAPTER 2:

The Occupational Safety & Health Administration site (OSHA) https://www.osha.gov/ SLTC/ formaldehyde/hazard_alert.html

Scientific American on children's study Phthalates http://www.scientificamerican.com/article. cfm?id=children-chemicals-fragrences-cosmetics-pthalate-attention-deficit-womb

Debra Lynn Dadd, **Home Safe Home** New York: Jeremy P. Tarcher/Putnam, 1997 p. 167–168.

Epstein, Samuel, M.D. (2001) **Unreasonable Risk**, Environmental Toxicology, Chicago, IL, 204 pp.

DeVita, S. (2014) **Vibrational Cleaning**, Tag Publishing, DeVita Wellness Institute, Can.

TIME Magazine (2002) July 15, July 22 editions, New York

CHAPTER 3:

Bharadwaj, Monisha (2000) **Indian Beauty Secrets**, Kyodo Printing Co., 160 pp.

Clark, Hulda (1999) **A Cure for All Advanced Cancer**, New Century Press

Colborn, T., Dumanoski, D. & Myers, J.P. (1997) **Our Stolen Future**, Penguin Books, New York, 316 pp.

Dr. Oz http://www.doctoroz.com/

Chopra, Deepak (1993) **Ageless Body, Timeless Mind**, Harmony Books, Crown Publishers, Inc.New York, 342 pp.

McTaggert, Lynn (1999) **"What Doctors Don't Tell You"** (WDDTY) Volume 10, #7 issue

Raichur, Pratima & Cohn, Marian (1997) **Absolute Beauty – Radiant Skin & Inner Harmony**, Harper Collins Publishers, Inc., New York, 421 pp.

Pert, Candace (1997) **"Molecules of Emotion"**, Touchstone, New York, NY. 368 pp.

Sachs, Melanie (1994) **Ayurvedic Beauty Care**, Lotus Press, Twin Lakes, WI. 285 pp.

Whitaker, J. & Colman, C. (1997) *Shed 10 Years In 10 Weeks*, Simon & Schuster, New York, 288 pp.

Dr. Bruce Lipton: *Biology of Belief*, Hay House, Inc, 2015

CHAPTER 4:

Andrew Weil, Dr. http://www.drweil.com

Borkovic, Joseph (2003) *"Know The Skin You're In"*, *Alive Magazine*, Alive Publishing Inc., Burnaby, BC, May Edition, page 92

Chopra, Deepak (2001) *"Grow Younger, Live Longer"*, Three Rivers Press, New York, 291 pp.

David Sinclair – http://www.hms.harvard.edu/agingresearch/index.php/about/staff/sinclair and *"When stem cells grow old: phenotypes and mechanisms of stem cell aging"*, 2016 Jan 1;143(1):3-14 https://www.ncbi.nlm.nih.gov/pubmed/26732838

https://www.youtube.com/watch?v=AiCvqnUle04 – You Tube

Raichur, Pratima & Cohn, Marian (1997) *"Absolute Beauty – Radiant Skin & Inner Harmony"*, Harper Collins Publishers, Inc., New York, 421 pp.

Somers, Suzanne, *"Bombshell"* 2012, Crown Publishing Group, Random House Inc. New York

Perricone, Nicholas (2000) *"The Wrinkle Cure"*, Rodale Reach, Rodale, U.S.A., 207 pp.

DeMarco, C. (1997) *"Take Charge of Your Body"*, The Well Women Press, Toronto, Canada, 295 pp. (Archives of Dermatology, January 2001; 137:53–59, 78–80)

Champagne http://www.columbia.edu/cu/psychology/fac-bios/ChampagneF/faculty.html http://steinhardt.nyu.edu/scmsAdmin/uploads/006/151/DP%20Champagne%20 2010.pdf

http://www.ucsf.edu/about/2009-nobel-prize-medicine/
elizabeth-blackburn-receives-nobel-prize-medicine

Adelle LaBrec —"*How to Reprogram Your DNA for Optimum Health*" 2014, Think Outside the Book Publishing, California

Vanderhaeghe, L. & Bouic, P. (1999) "*The Immune System Cure*", Prentice-Hall, Canada, Scarborough, Ontario, 250 pp.

Mitochondria http://www.mitoaction.org/blog/may-mito-meeting-drug-toxicity-mitochondria http://www.ncbi.nlm.nih.gov/pubmed/10961426 (http://www.nobelprize.org/nobel_prizes/medicine/laureates/2009 and http://biochemistry.ucsf.edu/labs/blackburn/index.php?Itemid=3)

Norm Shealy Dr. www.shealy.com

(http://www.telegraph.co.uk/news/science/science-news/11338225/Smartphones-and-tablets-cause-skin-wrinkling-condition-dubbed-tech-neck.html)

Lipton, Bruce Dr. "*The Biology of Belief*" Hay House, Inc, 2015

Childre, D. & Martin, H. (1999) "*The Heart Math Solution*", Harper Collins Publishers Inc.

Telomeres http://oracvalues.com/blog/telomere-length-telomerase-supplements-and-aging

Dr. Blackburn http://www.nobelprize.org/nobel_prizes/medicine/laureates/2009/blackburn-bio.html

Dr. Shealy https://normshealy.com

Dr. Christiane Northrup, 2015, "*Goddesses Never Age: The Secret Prescription for Radiance, Vitality, and Well-Being*" Hay House Inc.

Mental Health & Skin: http://www.mindbodygreen.com

Sheng R, Gu ZL, Xie ML. *Epigallocatechin gallate, the major component of polyphenols in green tea, inhibits telomere attrition mediated cariomyocyte apoptosis in cardiac hypertrophy.* Int J Cardiol. 2013 Jan 20;162(3):199–209. doi: 10.1016/j.ijcard.2011.07.083.

World Health Organization, *"Electromagnetic fields and public health: mobile phones."* Last modified

2011. *Accessed* March 27, 2013. http://www.who.int/mediacentre/factsheets/fs193/en/

Canada Newswire, *"Toronto Hospital is First to Recognize Symptoms from Wireless Radiation."* Last modified 2012. Accessed April 5, 2013. http://www.newswire.ca/en/story/994377/toronto-hospital-is-first-to-recognize-symptoms-from-wireless-radiation

Wilson, Bary. *"Evidence for an Effect of ELF Electromagnetic Fields on Human Pineal Gland Function."* Journal of Pineal Gland Research. 9. (1990): 259–269. http://efile.mpsc.state.mi.us/efile/docs/13934/0073.pdf (accessed April 5, 2013)

Poole, C. *"Depressive symptoms and headaches in relation to proximity of residence to an alternating-current transmission line right-of-way"* American Journal of Epidemiology. 137. no. 3 (1993): 318–330.

CHAPTER 5:

Goleman, Daniel (1997) *"Emotional Intelligence"*, Bantam Books, New York, NY, 352 pp.

Worwood, Valerie Ann (1990) *"The Fragrant Pharmacy"*, Bantam Books, Transworld Publishers, London, 546 pp.

Young, D. Gary (2000) *"A New Route to Robust Health"*, Essential Science Publishing, Salem, UT, 28 pp.

Damian, Peter & Kate (1995) *"Aromatherapy: Scent and Psyche"*, Healing Arts Press, Rochester,Vermont, 244 pp.

Stewart, David Ph.D. (2002) *"Healing Oils of the Bible"*, CARE Inc., Marble Hill, MO. 324 pp.

Penoél, Daniel & Rose-Marie (1998) "Natural Home Health Care Using Essential Oils" (translated, revised and enlarge from *"Pratique Aromatique Familiale"*, 1992, Brian Manwaring, editor, Essential Science Publishing, Orem, UT, 236 pp.

Raichur, Pratima & Cohn, Marian (1997) *"Absolute Beauty – Radiant Skin & Inner Harmony"*, Harper Collins Publishers, Inc., New York, 421 pp.

Pert, Candace (1997) *"Molecules of Emotion"*, Touchstone, New York, NY. 368 pp.

Whitaker, J. & Colman, C. (1997) *"Shed 10 Years In 10 Weeks"*, Simon & Schuster, New York, 288 pp.

Keville, Kathi (1999) *"Aromatherapy for Dummies"*, IDG Books Worldwide, Inc., Foster City, CA, 360 pp.

Whitaker, Julian (May 2002 and June 2002) *Health & Healing Newsletter*, Newport Beach, CA

CHAPTER 6:

Wilson, Roberta (2002) *"Aromatherapy: Essential Oils for Vibrant Health and Beauty"*, Avery-Penguin Putman Inc., New York. 340 pp.

Young, D. Gary (2002) *"Introduction to Essential Oils"*, tenth edition, Essential Oils Inc., Payson, UT, 140 pp.

Damian, Peter & Kate (1995) *"Aromatherapy: Scent and Psyche"*, Healing Arts Press, Rochester, Vermont, 244 pp.

Ramin Farzaneh-Far, M.D., of the University of California at San Francisco, lead author of *"Association of Marine Omega-3 Fatty Acid Levels with Telomeric Aging in Patients with Coronary Heart Disease"* JAMA 2010;303(3):250–257.

Dr. Mercola (http://articles.mercola.com/sites/articles/archive/2014/02/02/ketogenic-diet-health-benefits.aspx)

Lake, Rhody (2000) *"Liver Cleansing Handbook"*, Alive Books, Vancouver, BC, 62 pp. Manwaring, Brian, editor (2001) "Essential Oils Desk Reference", second edition, Essential Science Publishing, Orem, UT, 461 pp.

Stephanie Tourles, *"Naturally Healthy Skin"*, 1999 (Amazon.com)

David Wolfe, *'Eating for Beauty'*, 2003, (Amazon.com)

Dr. Jennifer Luke http://www.icnr.com/articles/fluoride-deposition.html

National Research Council. (2006). *Fluoride in Drinking Water: A Scientific Review of EPA's Standards* National Academies Press, Washington D.C

ZHANG Pengxia,LIANG Yunxia,TANG Xiaoli, et al. Authors address School of Basic Medical Science of Jiamusi University, Heilongjiang Jiamusi, 154007

Whitaker, J. & Colman, C. (1997) *"Shed 10 Years In 10 Weeks"*, Simon & Schuster, New York, 288 pp.

(Haroun, et al., 2002) Haroun, E.M., Mahmoud, O.M. & Adam, S.E. (2002) *Effect of feeding Cuminum cyminum fruits,Thymus vulgaris leaves or their mixture to rats.* Vet. Hum. Toxicol. Apr 44(2):67–9

Markus Rothkranz, 2011 Rothkranz Publishing, *"Heal Your Face"*

Dr. Oz http://www.doctoroz.com/article/dr-ozs-low-enzyme-test Dr. Oz- http://www.anewdayanewme.com/selenium

CHAPTER 8:

Moore, Neecie (1994) *"Boundless Health, Boundless Energy, Brilliant Youth: The Truth About DHEA"*, Claris Publishing Co. Inc., Texas, 179 pp.

Colborn, T., Dumanoski, D. & Myers, J.P. (1997) "Our Stolen Future", Penguin Books, New York, 316 pp.

Young, D. Gary (2000) *"Pregnenolone"*, Essential Science Publishing, Utah, 63 pp.

Dr. Brownstein, http://www.brownstein.com

Berg, Eric, D.C. (2001) *"Healthy Hormones, Healthy Life"*, Health & Wellness Center, Virginia 86 pp. http://www.icnr.com/articles/fluoride-deposition.html

National Research Council 2006

Whitaker, Julian (May 2002 and June 2002) *Health & Healing Newsletter*, Newport Beach, CA

DeVita, S. (2000) *"Electromagnetic Pollution"*, Stewart Publishing Company, Missouri, U.S., 84 pp.

CHAPTER 9:

Jamieson & Dorman *"The Role of Somatotroph – Specific Peptides and IGF-1 Intermediates as an Alternative to HGH Injections"* by James Jamieson & L.E.

Dorman, D.R., presented for the American College for Advancement in Medicine, October 30, 1997.

Journal of the American College of Nutrition, 2001: 20:71 – 80

Young, D. Gary (2014) "Einkorn", Life Sciences Publishing, Utah, *"Fats that Heal and Fats that Kill"*, Udo Erasmus

Chia – (http://www.happyhealthylonglife.com/happy_healthy_long_life/2008/07/are-the-chia-pet-seeds-salvia-hispanica-the-new-improved-flax-seed.html)

Sea Buckthorn http://articles.mercola.com/herbal-oils/sea-buckthorn-oil.aspx Sea Buckthorn, http://www.chatelaine.com/health/wellness/seabuckthorn

Resveratrol http://www.mayoclinic.org/diseases-conditions/heart-disease/in-depth/red-wine/art-20048281

Curry consumption and cognitive function in the elderly http://www.ncbi.nlm.nih.gov/pubmed/16870699

Doherty, B. & Van Tine, Julia (2002) *"Growing Younger"*, Rodale, Rodale Inc., U.S.A., 404 pp.

Dr. Eve Cauter Lancet, 1999

Dr. Andrew Weil http://www.drweil.com

CHAPTER 10:

Haroun, E.M., Mahmoud, O.M. & Adam, S.E. (2002) *Effect of feeding Cuminum cyminum fruits, Thymus vulgaris leaves or their mixture to rats*. Vet. Hum. Toxicol. Apr 44(2):67–9

Mercola, Joseph D.O. http://articles.mercola.com/herbal-oils/clary-sage-oil.aspx

Mercola, Joseph D.O. http://articles.mercola.com/herbal-oils/bergamot-oil.aspx

Worwood, Valerie Ann (1990) *"The Fragrant Pharmacy"*, Bantam Books, Transworld Publishers, London, 546 pp.

Wilson, Roberta (2002) *"Aromatherapy: Essential Oils for Vibrant Health and Beauty"*, Avery-Penguin Putman Inc., New York. 340 pp.

CHAPTER 11:

Bharadwaj, Monisha (2000) *"Indian Beauty Secrets"*, Kyodo Printing Co., 160 pp.

Young, D. Gary (2002) *"Introduction to Essential Oils"*, tenth edition, Essential Oils Inc., Payson, UT, 140 pp.

Worwood, Valerie Ann (1990) *"The Fragrant Pharmacy"*, Bantam Books, Transworld Publishers, London, 546 pp.

Raichur, Pratima & Cohn, Marian (1997) *"Absolute Beauty – Radiant Skin & Inner Harmony"*, Harper Collins Publishers, Inc., New York, 421 pp.

Schnaubelt, Kurt (1995) *"Advanced Aromatherapy"*, Healing Arts Press Rochester, Vermont, 138 pp.

Life Science Publishing (2011) *"Essential Oils Desk Reference"* Special fifth edition, Life Science Publishers

CHAPTER 12:

Wesley-Hosford, Zia (1983) *"Being Beautiful"*, Fine Design Book Works, Mill Valley, CA, 187 pp.

Kushi, Michio (1981) *"Oriental Diagnosis: What Your Face Reveals"*, Sunwheel Publication, London, 80pp.

Husain, Shahnaz (1998) *"Shahnaz Husain's Beauty Book"*, Orient Paperbacks, Delhi, India, 183 pp.

Johnson, Anne (2001) *"The Body Book"*, Klutz Inc., Palo Alto, CA, 67 pp.

Turmeric – http://www.turmericforhealth.com/turmeric-cures/turmeric-masks-for-great-skin#ixzz3Pnuhm5Su

Dennison, Paul E. Ph. D. (1986) *"Brain Gym"*, Edu-Kinesthetics, Inc., Ventura, CA, 41 pp.

Gerber, R. (1988) *"Vibrational Medicine"*, Bear & Company, Santa Fe, NM, 559 pp.

Tolle, Eckhart (1999) *"The Power of Now"*, Namaste Publishing Inc., Canada, 191 pp.

CHAPTER 13:

Ortner, Nick (2013) *"The Tapping Solution: A Revolutionary System For Stress-Free Living"*, Hay House Publishing, United States

Almine, (2010) *"Secrets of Rejuvenation"*, Spiritual Journeys, Newport, Oregon

DeVita, Sabina (2010) *"Emotional Freedom Face-Lift"*, Sound Concepts, U.S.

RESOURCES:

Energy Technologies: www.devitawellnessclinics.weebly.com

GDV Bio-electrography (Kirlian): Geoffrey Riley, & Dr. Sabina DeVita, www.b-wellnow.net

Young Living Essential Oils: 1–800–371–3515 (a sponsor member name/number is required as a customer or as a member)

Synova Derma – Allergy Research Group: **1–800–545–9960**

Toki – Lane Labs: **1–866–510–2010**

ABOUT THE AUTHOR

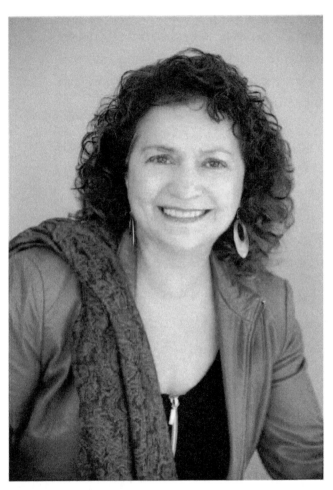

Sabina M. DeVita (Ed.D, N.N.C.P., IASP, CBP,) has been a long time environmentalist. When she became ill in the 1980's, with environmental sensitivities, also known as ecological illness or multiple chemical sensitivities (MCS), she was forced to change her life path dramatically. She experienced many ill effects physically, mentally and emotionally from environmental and chemical sensitivities. She left her position as a teacher then guidance counselor of many years in the public school system to pursue her doctoral interests in psychology and environmental sensitivities due to her illness. Her doctoral dissertation on brain allergies and mental health issues, a rare combination not at all known or considered even to this day became the first work of its kind in the field of psychology at the University of Toronto as well as in environmental & ecological sensitivities. With her pioneering spirit, she completed her doctoral dissertation in 1986 on 'Cerebral Allergies, An Understanding of the Phenomenon and Its Psychological Implications'—an understanding of Body, Mind and Spirit.

In the late 90's she discovered the power of real, organic, therapeutic grade A essential oils and the art & science of French medicinal aromatherapy. She became involved with the company that is considered today as the World Leader in Essential oils, the "Seed to Seal" Young Living company. These precious and live-food essential oils were introduced into her practices and in all of her classes as a powerful solution to many of humanity's health, beauty, mental and physical needs along with her energy dowsing and kinesiology techniques.

She is certified as a Registered Nutritional coach-consultant as well as in Holistic Energy Psychology and Essential oils sciences, Egyptian dowsing and specialized Kinesiology and Body Talk. She is Director and Founder of the DeVita Wellness Institute of Living and Learning with 27 years as an eclectic psychotherapist.

She is also Director—Founder of the federally approved **Institute of Energy Wellness Studies** of the last 7 years. Dr. DeVita is an accomplished author of six books with her most popular book: *"Vibrational Cleaning"* and its sequel that has gained international recognition. She is an international speaker/instructor, featured in the documentary film called: The Wellness Story along with several Rogers TV programs and radio interviews on her latest books. She was trained by D. Gary Young founder of Young Living Essential Oils with over 850 hours in essential oil sciences information along with application and certified by Gary in 2007 as a Raindrop technique Instructor.

Dr. DeVita is certified in Russia as a GDV Kirlian Bio-electrographic practitioner and instructor by the inventor scientist, physicist, Dr. K. Korotkov. She holds Grand master in Belvaspata. She is a graduate from the Bio-Geometry program on the physics of quality with both Dr. Robert Gilbert and Dr. Ibrahim Karim (founder of Bio-Geometry) and incorporates some of the simple Bio-Geometry principles (www.bgwellnessnow.com) into her writings with further plans to help educate many more with her teaching the virtues of utilizing Bio-Geometry into their lives.

CPSIA information can be obtained
at www.ICGtesting.com
Printed in the USA
LVOW05s0718040517
533044LV00007B/3/P